W0018414

Framing Global Health Governance

This edited collection looks at how globalisation is influencing patterns of health and disease worldwide, in particular how decisions on health are made and organised.

Despite some successes in developing better global governance for health, overall progress has been disappointingly slow given the number of health crises today, both long standing and relatively new. This book explores how progress has often been limited, but also on occasion assisted, by the role of ideas. It identifies how health issues, such as HIV/AIDS, pandemic influenza and tobacco control, are framed in such a way as to resonate with a set of ideas, or worldviews, associated with particular policy communities. A successful framing can generate possibilities for action, but can also lead to competition when ideas conflict or suggest different pathways of response. Global Health Governance is therefore an arena of competition as well as cooperation, where ideas matter as well as resources and political will.

This book was originally published as a special issue of *Global Public Health*.

Colin McInnes is the UNESCO Chair in HIV/AIDS Education and Health Security in Africa and Director of the Centre for Health and International Relations at Aberystwyth University, UK.

Kelley Lee is a Professor in the Faculty of Health Sciences and Director of Global Health at Simon Fraser University, Canada.

Framing Global Health Governance

Edited by
Colin McInnes and Kelley Lee

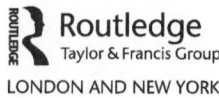
Routledge
Taylor & Francis Group

LONDON AND NEW YORK

First published in paperback 2024

First published 2015
by Routledge
4 Park Square, Milton Park, Abingdon, Oxon OX14 4RN

and by Routledge
605 Third Avenue, New York, NY 10158

Routledge is an imprint of the Taylor & Francis Group, an informa business

© 2015, 2024 Taylor & Francis

All rights reserved. No part of this book may be reprinted or reproduced or utilised in any form or by any electronic, mechanical, or other means, now known or hereafter invented, including photocopying and recording, or in any information storage or retrieval system, without permission in writing from the publishers.

Trademark notice: Product or corporate names may be trademarks or registered trademarks, and are used only for identification and explanation without intent to infringe.

Publisher's Note
The publisher has gone to great lengths to ensure the quality of this reprint but points out that some imperfections in the original copies may be apparent.

Disclaimer
Every effort has been made to contact copyright holders for their permission to reprint material in this book. The publishers would be grateful to hear from any copyright holder who is not here acknowledged and will undertake to rectify any errors or omissions in future editions of this book.

British Library Cataloguing in Publication Data
A catalogue record for this book is available from the British Library

ISBN: 978-1-138-78800-8 (hbk)
ISBN: 978-1-03-293063-3 (pbk)
ISBN: 978-1-315-76571-6 (ebk)

DOI: 10.4324/9781315765716

Typeset in Times New Roman
by Taylor & Francis Books

Contents

Citation Information

The chapters in this book were originally published in *Global Public Health*, volume 7, Supplement 2 (December 2012). When citing this material, please use the original page numbering for each article, as follows:

Chapter 7

Making a human right to tobacco control: Expert and advocacy networks, framing and the right to health
David Reubi
Global Public Health, volume 7, issue 2 (December 2012) pp. S176–S190

Chapter 8

Framing and global health governance: Key findings
Colin McInnes and Kelley Lee
Global Public Health, volume 7, issue 2 (December 2012) pp. S191–S198

Please direct any queries you may have about the citations to
clsuk.permissions@cengage.com

Notes on Contributors

Adam Kamradt-Scott, Centre for International Security Studies (CIIS), University of Sydney, Sydney, Australia

Kelley Lee, Department of Global Health and Development, Faculty of Public Health and Policy, London School of Hygiene and Tropical Medicine (LSHTM), London, UK and Faculty of Health Sciences, Simon Fraser University, Burnaby, Canada

Colin McInnes, Department of International Politics, Centre for Health and International Relations (CHAIR), Aberystwyth University, Aberystwyth, UK

David Reubi, Department of Global Health and Development, Faculty of Public Health and Policy, London School of Hygiene and Tropical Medicine (LSHTM), London, UK and Centre for International Security Studies (CIIS), University of Sydney, Sydney, Australia

Anne Roemer-Mahler, Department of Global Health and Development, Faculty of Public Health and Policy, London School of Hygiene and Tropical Medicine (LSHTM), London, UK

Simon Rushton, Department of Politics, University of Sheffield, Sheffield, UK

Owain David Williams, Consultant on Global Health

Marie Woodling, Department of International Politics, Centre for Health and International Relations (CHAIR), Aberystwyth University, Aberystwyth, UK

INTRODUCTION

Framing global health: The governance challenge

Colin McInnes[a], Adam Kamradt-Scott[c], Kelley Lee[b,d], David Reubi[b,e], Anne Roemer-Mahler[b], Simon Rushton[a], Owain David Williams[a] and Marie Woodling[a]

[a]*Department of International Politics, Centre for Health and International Relations (CHAIR), Aberystwyth University, Aberystwyth, UK;* [b]*Department of Global Health and Development, Faculty of Public Health and Policy, London School of Hygiene and Tropical Medicine (LSHTM), London, UK;* [c]*Centre for International Security Studies (CIIS), University of Sydney, Sydney, Australia;* [d]*Faculty of Health Sciences, Simon Fraser University, Burnaby, Canada;* [e]*School of Global Studies, University of Sussex, Brighton, UK*

With the emergence of global health comes governance challenges which are equally global in nature. This article identifies some of the initial limitations in analyses of global health governance (GHG) before discussing the focus of this special supplement: the framing of global health issues and the manner in which this impacts upon GHG. Whilst not denying the importance of material factors (such as resources and institutional competencies), the article identifies how issues can be framed in different ways, thereby creating particular pathways of response which in turn affect the potential for and nature of GHG. It also identifies and discusses the key frames operating in global health: evidence-based medicine, human rights, security, economics and development.

Globalisation is widely seen as influencing patterns of health and disease worldwide (Dodgson *et al.* 2002, Cockerham and Cockerham 2010, McInnes and Lee, 2012). It is also understood as both causing and requiring changes to how decisions on health policy are made and organised. It has caused change, not least through the emergence of new bodies with global reach. It requires change because if 'health is global' (DoH 2008), then collective solutions are required for shared health problems. Thus the emergence of 'global heath governance' (GHG) is widely seen in two ways. First, it is seen in terms of institutional developments – the emergence of new global actors such as the GAVI Alliance; the Global Fund to Fight HIV/AIDS, Tuberculosis and Malaria (GFATM) and the Bill and Melinda Gates Foundation (Ollila 2005, Buse *et al.* 2009, Williams and Rushton 2011), or the adoption of new roles and responsibilities by the existing actors such as the WHO or the World Bank (Dodgson *et al.* 2002, Ruger 2005, Cockerham and Cockerham 2010). Second, the emergence of GHG is also seen in an ostensibly rationalist light as a reasoned response to an exogenous development, namely the globalisation of health determinants and outcomes (Collin *et al.* 2002, Fidler 2004).

Both the nature of emerging global health problems and the necessary mechanisms of GHG to deal with them, however, have historically been narrowly defined in both the policy and academic worlds (although more recently movement to broaden this focus has been apparent[1]). In particular, four limitations can be identified through much of the available policy and academic literature:

- The existing analysis has emphasised the institutional and technical features of GHG actors and policies, and has failed to adequately grasp more fundamental reasons for the disjuncture between global health needs and governance responses (see Kay and Williams 2009).
- Research so far has with some success analysed individual global health institutions or mechanisms, but there has been little comparative analysis to draw wider lessons for strengthening GHG (see Youde 2012).
- Analysis to date has focused heavily on infectious diseases and SARS, HIV/AIDS and pandemic influenza in particular (Fidler 2004, 2010, Davies 2008). Although vitally important, limited attention has been given to the governance challenges posed by the wider range of global health issues faced.
- Attention has focused on material factors such as disease outbreaks, funding mechanisms and preparedness plans. Only comparatively recently have ideational factors – the ideas that shape our understanding of issues, thereby creating acceptable pathways of response – begun to be examined (see Shiffman 2009).

These limitations led to the establishment in January 2009 of a four-year project examining competing visions of GHG, funded by the European Research Council, involving a multidisciplinary team co-located at the Centre for Health and International Relations at Aberystwyth University (CHAIR) as well as the Centre on Global Change and Health in the Department of Global Health and Development at the London School of Hygiene and Tropical Medicine (LSHTM). The project's aim has been to look beyond institutional (in)competencies and technical responses; to broaden the focus to understand a broad range of global health challenges; to examine the ways in which responses to global health crises are shaped by a contested space of competing ideas and worldviews of health; and to offer a comparative analysis across a range of health issues.

This special supplement of *Global Public Health* considers the way in which GHG has been influenced by the world of ideas. To facilitate this, the supplement adopts a constructivist theoretical approach, which allows an examination of the ideational as well as material basis behind contemporary debates and controversies. As Onuf (1989) argues, the social world is one of our own making where the ideas we use shape our understanding of that world. This does not mean that the material world is of no concern, but rather that the material and ideational interact with each other:

'Constructivists hold the view that the building blocks of . . . reality are ideational as well as material; that ideational factors have normative as well as instrumental dimensions; that they express not only individual but collective intentionality; and that the meaning and significance of ideational factors are not independent of time and place' (Ruggie 1998, p. 33).

Therefore, in this collection we do not deny the importance of material factors in shaping GHG, but add to this the manner in which health and health issues are socially constructed (by language and other means) and *through this construction* possess meaning. Specifically, we use ideas of 'framing', whereby an issue is presented in such a way as to tie it into a broader set of ideas about the world, or 'socially constructed reality', and through this gain influence and policy purchase. Frames are defined by Gitlin as 'persistent patterns of cognition, interpretation and presentation, of selection, emphasis and exclusion, by which symbol-handlers routinely organise discourse' (1980, p. 7). Framing has been used extensively in the public policy literature (see Entman 1993, Fischer 2003, Jerit 2008), though perhaps less so in public health (see Dorfman and Woodruff 2005) and only recently in a very limited number of studies pertaining to GHG (Shiffman 2009, Labonté and Gagnon 2010). In policy debates, actors often deliberately (and in many cases strategically) use frames as a tool of persuasion, deploying them to call attention to an issue, influence other actors' perceptions of their own interests and convince them of the legitimacy/ appropriateness of the advocate's preferred policy response. When they are successful in doing so, the chosen frame 'resonates with public understandings, and are adopted as new ways of talking about and understanding issues', and actors will be likely to modify their behaviour accordingly (Finnemore and Sikkink 1998, p. 897).

Frames are deployed and promoted by various stakeholders, including transnational advocacy groups, international organisations and epistemic communities. These are the 'cognitive baggage handlers of constructivist analyses' (Haas 1992 cited in Youde 2005, p. 423). In global public health, competing 'baggage handlers' frame health issues in particular ways (as a biomedical, human rights, security or economic issue), in an attempt to generate or legitimise specific pathways of response on health issues. For example, in this collection, Kamradt-Scott and McInnes (2012) point out how pandemic influenza has been framed as a security issue (or 'threat') to generate support for emergency plans and preparation, while Reubi identifies how a network of activists successfully framed tobacco control as a human rights issue in order to tie it into the existing legislation on human rights. Not all of these 'baggage handlers' are equal, but they have differential power, including intangible factors such as social capital, which can lead to one group being more successful than another. But framings can also be constitutive of meaning – that is, they may move beyond being merely a presentational artifice to become a means of shaping the way in which a health issue is understood. They achieve this by presenting an issue in terms that have meaning for a worldview and therefore are associative with that worldview. Thus, to follow the earlier example, framing pandemic influenza as a security issue has led not only to action being undertaken on the issue, but also to the very nature of the disease being understood in terms of posing a 'threat'. What may therefore begin as a political tactic to gain attention and resources for a health issue may become central to the construction of its meaning. Therefore, in this collection we use the fruits of an ongoing four-year multidisciplinary research programme to examine the manner in which health issues are framed, for what purposes and with what effects.

It should be noted from the outset that global *governance* is defined here as conceptually distinct from global *government*. The focus of global governance is not on the creation of a supranational authority with the legitimacy to impose globally binding laws and regulations over states' wishes. Nor is it solely concerned with formal agreements or arrangements such as treaties, convention regulations or international institutions, though in much of the literature on GHG, these remain the general focus of attention. Instead, it covers a range of formal and informal agreements, principles and understandings that inform acceptable behaviour. Governance may indeed be formal, and may involve relinquishing sovereignty in particular circumstances, but it may also be seen in tacit agreements, informal understandings and the positional power of organisations and institutions (see Rosenau and Czempiel 1992, Rosenau 1995, Hewson and Sinclair 1999). It therefore covers a wide spectrum of possibilities and accepts that those involved may include not only traditional actors such as states and international institutions, but also global civil society and charitable foundations. Nor is it necessarily the case that formal agreements such as treaties and conventions, which are ostensibly binding in terms of international law, are necessarily more important to GHG than tacit agreements or shared understandings: a treaty with no monitoring or enforcement mechanisms may not be honoured, while a widely accepted understanding of what should be done under certain circumstances may prove much more significant in governing behaviour.

The key advantage in using framing to understand and explain GHG, then, is its introduction of an ideational element: how the manner in which a health issue is framed opens up specific acceptable pathways of governance response based upon shared understandings (or what is sometimes referred to as 'worldviews'). How issues are framed can tap into powerful ideational forces that may prove as significant as institutional competencies, interests and agendas in shaping GHG, including creating difficulties for effective GHG.

Project background

The core challenge for GHG is how collective action on an increasingly broad range of shared global health concerns can be more effectively achieved. We have already detailed some of our concerns over the generally narrow focus of much of the literature. The attempt to embed a broadened conception of what GHG encompasses is therefore a key component of this project. But the project is also underpinned by an understanding that the challenge of GHG is not simply technical – of devising appropriate institutional configurations and competencies and treatment regimes – but a political one. By this we mean that the sort of problems encountered in GHG are not amenable to rational, value-neutral analysis leading to an optimal solution, but exist in an arena where different values, interests and knowledge create competition and contestation. GHG is inherently political because it raises fundamental questions regarding where power and authority does and should lie in governing to protect and promote human health, and whose interests should be served or not served by the distribution of costs and benefits arising from such authority. For example, access to antiviral drugs during an influenza pandemic raises the question of how to balance national interests and those of the global commons. This is an inherently political question, but so is that of who has the authority to make a decision on this and similar global health issues. This is one of the reasons why GHG has developed into a highly contested space. But the space is also contested because there is no single underlying logic behind calls for action. Rather, there are a variety of presentational artifices that have been used to gain attention to different (and sometimes the same) health issues, each of which may suggest a particular pathway of policy response underpinned by a particular governance framework. Thus, and rather simplistically, framing pandemic influenza as a security threat is likely to privilege national over collective regional or global interests, to suggest a territorially focused policy of 'at the border' controls and to promote disease surveillance as a core GHG response. In contrast, framing influenza as a development issue is informed by the idea of a shared humanity where rights and responsibilities are couched more widely; it may suggest policies that focus on upstream causes of disease, including levels of poverty, and would involve the provision of aid for capacity building in the GHG responses. The project's framing approach, therefore, helps us to understand how GHG is shaped by different, and at times competing, perspectives and worldviews of the nature and causes of global health problems and the appropriate solutions to them. The articles in this special supplement demonstrate how the framing of global health issues and their associated governance responses to date have led to the creation of particular pathways of response. Moreover, like Shiffman (2009) we are interested not only in advancing our understanding of how certain framings may prove more persuasive and expedient than others in generating action on global health issues, but also how action may be constrained by competing framings that may cross institutional boundaries.

Research design and methods

An initial scoping study supported our hypothesis that there was little by way of comparative analysis in GHG, and that much of the literature focused on the problem of infectious disease. From the start, therefore, the project has been designed around four comparative case studies that form the empirical basis of the articles that follow. These include not only infectious diseases as key generators of discussion on GHG (for this project we use HIV/AIDS and pandemic influenza as case studies), but also non-communicable disease (tobacco control) and distributive issues (access to medicines). To facilitate comparison across case studies, we adopted a standard 'structured focused' methodology (George 1979). The temporal focus starting in the 1990s was chosen because it marked major changes in both the international system and in Development Assistance for Health (DAH). It is also the period when health began to be constructed as being global (Brown et al. 2006). A second scoping study identified five key frames to be examined across the case studies: biomedicine, security, development, economics and human rights. These frames were not unique to the case studies examined by this project, but appeared to be dominant framings across the emerging realm of global health. However, subsequent work led us to modify this approach in two important respects. First, biomedicine proved an unwieldy frame to operationalise and research, and a narrower but related frame of 'evidence-based medicine' (EBM) was focused upon given the impact of this movement on biomedical research and policy over the past 20 years. Second, we had an initial concern that most of the frames were internally contested, with competing theories, methodologies and approaches leading to different policy prescriptions, making their value as frames uncertain. In this respect, EBM perhaps suffered the least, but each of the others appeared to a greater or lesser extent to be potentially problematic. We needed to identify a higher-level commonality in worldview that defined the frame as coherent although internal contestations could still be acknowledged. This is reflected in the brief introductions to the frames used later in this paper and in several of the papers in this collection, including those by Reubi (2012), by Williams (2012) and by Woodling *et al.* (2012). A crucial move was to accept that the identification of specific frames as coherent was to some extent heuristic in that it simplified reality for analytical purposes, but in a nonetheless useful manner. Further empirical research has subsequently supported our scoping study in that, although other frames might exist, these five have been dominant in global health and, in particular, GHG.

The research used available primary and secondary literature and key informant interviews. Literature was identified using keyword searches on online databases (including Google Scholar, ISI Web of Knowledge, JSTOR, LexisNexis, OCLC ArticleFirst and PubMed), with further sources cascading from these. Texts included scholarly works, 'grey' literature and policy papers. Following a review of the literature, we were able to produce a 'spotter's guide' of key features for each of the frames under analysis prior to the first phase of interviewing. For each frame we identified the following: knowledge, arguments and language used; the communities of experts involved; and techniques (or what some might term 'technologies') of governance. These were not intended to be binding and inflexible tools, but rather to provide a common understanding across the case studies, enabling us to identify the operation and influence of frames. The 'spotter's guides' were consequently amenable to review as further data were received. During 2010 and 2011, over 300 interviews were conducted in locations including Atlanta, Bangkok, Brussels, Canberra, Geneva, London, Manila, Nairobi, New York, Singapore and Washington DC, with policy-makers, government officials, civil servants (including staff at international organisations), civil society and academia. Interviews were semi-structured using a data bank of questions common across the case studies. The interviews were digitally recorded, transcribed and shared through a secure SharePoint site. As approved by the Research Ethics Committees of both the LSHTM and Aberystwyth University, all interviews were conducted on a confidential basis unless the key informant agreed otherwise. The interviews have been used extensively to support the following papers, but for these reasons of confidentiality we have omitted reference to them (unless the interview subjects gave prior permission) and used published sources wherever possible.

Frames

This section briefly introduces the five frames used by the project and reflected in this collection. As already noted, these are heuristic devices that we use as analytical tools while simultaneously recognising the presence of internal contestations in many of these frames and their potential.

EBM initially gained prominence in the mid-1990s, but by 1998 the movement had spread rapidly internationally to become fully embedded within the majority of medical (clinical) training programmes. At its core, EBM encourages and reinforces positivist, rationalist ways of reasoning – namely, that a world exists independent of observation that can be analysed using epidemiological and biostatistical tools to provide data that will inform health-related policy decisions (see Davidoff *et al.* 1995,

Rosenberg and Donald 1995, Sackett *et al.* 1995, 1996). As a direct result of its integration into contemporary training programmes, successive generations of medical/clinical practitioners have been trained in EBM methods and ways of thinking. As a result, EBM has become the primary mode of scientific, rational enquiry for contemporary biomedicine and clinical practice and the key frame for the health policy community (Tonelli 1998, Kristiansen and Mooney 2004). Use of this frame is often identifiable by reference to 'evidence' to support decision-making and the deployment of particular techniques such as 'systematic reviews' to inform policy development. In this regard, language is strategic in that the adoption and use of terms such as 'evidence based' and 'systematic' reify and reinforce rationalist thinking while simultaneously categorising and condemning other forms of reasoning as inferior (i.e., who would not want to use evidence to support their decision-making? Who would not wish to be systematic?).

Over the past 20 years, there has been a marked resurgence in framing global public health issues in terms of *human rights* (see Reubi 2012). Perhaps the two most significant issues in this resurgence were HIV/AIDS and, later, access to medicines (Olesen 2006, Biehl *et al.* 2009, Rushton, 2012). However, other global health issues have also been framed as human rights problems, from maternal and child health to tobacco control (Shiffman and Smith 2007, Reubi 2012), while from the late 1980s/early 1990s, the gradual shift from population to reproductive health also contributed significantly to the prioritisation of human rights in global health. Unsurprisingly, the relationship between the moral-legal rhetoric of human rights and global health is highly contested. Indeed, even within a same organisation there can be competing understandings of how human rights and health relate. One can, however, still identify understandings that have been particularly influential over the last two decades. One of these is that developed initially in the 1990s by Jonathan Mann (the former Director of the World Health Organization's Global Programme on AIDS) and subsequently developed by other AIDS advocates (Fee and Parry 2008). For them, human rights are moral values that should guide public health experts and ensure that their policies and practices are not discriminatory, coercive or undemocratic (see Mann *et al.* 1994, 1999). Another influential understanding of human rights and health is that which developed during the twenty-first century by both the UN Committee on Economic, Social and Cultural Rights (UNCESCR) and the UN Special Rapporteur on the Right to Health, Paul Hunt. For them, the relationship between human rights and health is primarily about the right to health: the right to receive appropriate and affordable health care (see UNCESCR 2000, Hunt 2004, Hunt and Backman 2008). Unlike Mann's definition, this conception of human rights and health emphasised the importance of international legal norms like article 12 of the 1966 International Covenant on Economic, Social and Cultural Rights (IESCR), judicial enforcement mechanisms and human rights lawyers (Reubi 2012).

Economics is a particularly diverse and internally contested frame (Amariglio 1990). Health economics, by extension, is no exception. For example, market-based theories (that supply is best determined by demand, and price is best set by a 'free' market) compete with public-goods theories (that public provision of health is rational because of the innate qualities of health and its contribution to economic growth). Each theory, however, infers a rational basis of how to use and distribute scarce resources, and it is this which underpins economic framings of health. The basic underlying logic that unites all variants of economics in the context of health is that demand for health is inelastic (if you are ill then your demand for treatment does not vary with your income or the price of the treatment), and that the resources that can be devoted to health are scarce. The economic frame is therefore manifested when arguments about efficiency, choice and competitiveness are used to justify the distribution of these scarce resources in particular ways. Thus, health economics is about the rational basis for making choices regarding how to deploy and distribute scarce resources to optimally meet health needs (see Mills 1997) and generally employs the methodology of classical liberal economics (e.g., cost–benefit analysis).

Like economics, *security* is highly contested. Traditionally, security has been narrowly understood in terms of a clear and present danger to the state, but over the past two decades this has broadened to include other referent objects and a wider range of risks, some of which may be more tangible than others (Buzan 2001, Booth 2007). This led Buzan to suggest that security is 'essentially contested' (see Booth 2007, p. 99) – that is, a concept which generates unsolvable debates about its meaning and application. These contestations have allowed a variety of different terms to become used in the framing of health security, each implying different referent objects (i.e., whose security should be protected). These include human security, national security, international security and global health security. The underlying logic that is common to all forms of security, however, is that of threat and defence (see Gray 2009), though sometimes alternative terms such as 'risk' and 'protection' might be used (see Williams 2009). Thus, health becomes a security issue when it is perceived and presented in the following ways: (1) as a threat to someone or something and (2) as something which defensive measures (either in the form of prevention or response) must be taken against. This is the hallmark of the security frame in global health: x is a threat/risk to a referent object in respect to which we must put defensive/protective measures y in place.

As with the previous two frames, *development* is contested, with multiple meanings. Although there is no single, universally applicable narrative of development, most proponents share an enthusiasm to improve conditions and establish progress in the Third World, where the First World becomes something of a benchmark for measurement (for a critical perspective on this, see Escobar 1995, 2004). The ultimate goal of improving (health in) the Third World is presented as unarguable and a universal given; rather, the means to achieve it form the point of disagreement for advocates, with a plethora of theories such as modernisation, dependency and trickle-down economics going in and out of fashion (recent examples of this include Farmer 2003, Sachs 2005, Collier 2007). Development narratives are characterised by a series of hierarchical binaries (developed/underdeveloped, donor/ recipient, rich/poor, healthy/unhealthy, active/passive, hegemonic/subordinate, strong/weak, etc.), which place the idea of 'lack' vis-à-vis the developed world at the heart of this frame (Escobar 1995, 2004). But development is a problematic frame: it seems that health in the Third World must *always* be a matter for development, although other frames/paradigms will most probably also play a part.

Conclusion

The following articles are therefore based upon a coherent research programme examining the contested realm of GHG. This collection focuses on the ideational realm – the ideas that shape the field in both policy and academic terms. Specifically, these articles examine the manner in which health issues are framed, for what purpose and with what effects. Each of the following articles uses one of the five frames previously identified in this paper as being dominant in GHG, to examine one of the four case studies used by the project. Comparison is possible for two of the case studies (HIV/AIDS and pandemic influenza), with both being examined by different frames, and two different frames (security and development) being used to examine the same issue. Kamradt-Scott explores the influence of EBM on pandemic influenza preparedness, and how vaccines and antiviral medicines are promoted as indicators of pandemic preparedness. In particular, he notes how EBM has further reinforced the advocacy of drug-based solutions, placing vaccines and then antivirals centre stage while downplaying alternative preparedness measures. Reubi addresses the recent proliferation of human rights approaches in public health by focusing on the issue of tobacco control. Crucially, he shows how framing can be used not simply to generate attention for an issue but how, by reframing tobacco control as a human rights issue, the existing legislation on human rights could then be brought to bear on tobacco control. Reubi also demonstrates how a small but influential network can succeed in reframing an issue. Williams identifies how the patent system has been framed in economic terms as necessary or even benign in establishing a system that allows new drugs to be developed and traded; he finds that this has created a range of difficulties for access to medicines and ultimately a dysfunctional global drug market. Despite the emergence of a range of new actors intent on broadening access by intervening on drug price and innovation, Williams remains sceptical of their impact, given the strength of the economic framing of the patent/trade regime. The security frame is considered in two articles. Rushton examines the debate over limitations imposed on HIV-positive travellers in light of the US decision in 2010 to repeal its legislation. Restrictions had been imposed using a security frame, while opponents of the legislation attempted to undermine this framing by challenging the empirical evidence or by counter-framing it as a human rights issue. Rushton concludes that the counter-framing proved insufficient in itself to change US policy and that other factors, including changing political context and network building strategies by opponents to the legislation, were necessary factors. In the second article using the security frame, Kamradt-Scott and McInnes use the Copenhagen School's securitisation theory to examine how pandemic influenza has been framed as a security issue. They conclude that the act of framing was insufficient on its own, and that material factors (especially disease outbreaks such as SARS and H1N1) were necessary for a successful securitisation. But once securitisation had occurred, it then proved effective in driving policy change. Finally, Woodling, Williams and Rushton argue that although HIV/AIDS has been framed in a number of different ways, thereby allowing a multisectoral approach to emerge, development has proved a particularly powerful and resilient frame. This has been seen recently when, with other health issues beginning to claim attention away from HIV/AIDS, the development frame was used in an attempt to re-establish AIDS' special status.

Acknowledgements

This research has been made possible through funding from the European Research Council under the European Community's Seventh Framework Programme – Ideas Grant 230489 GHG. All views expressed remain those of the authors.

Note

1. Not least in the policy world, where maternal health care featured prominently in both the 2010 UN summit on the Millennium Development Goals (MDGs) and the G8 meeting of the same year. In 2011 the UN held a summit on non-communicable diseases (NCDs).

References

Amariglio, J., 1990. *Economics as a discourse*. Boston: Kluwer.

Biehl, J., Petryna, A., Gertner, A., Amon, J., and Picon, P., 2009. Judicialisation of the right to health in Brazil. *The Lancet*, 373, 2182–2184.

Booth, K., 2007. *Theory of world security*. Cambridge: Cambridge University Press.

Brown, T.M., Cuerte, M., and Fee, E., 2006. The World Health Organization and the transition from international to global public health. *American Journal of Public Health*, 96 (1), 62–72.

Buse, K., Hein, W., and Drager, N., eds. 2009. *Making sense of global health governance: a policy perspective*. Basingstoke: Palgrave Macmillan.

Buzan, B., 2001. *People, states, and fear: an agenda for international security studies in the post-Cold War era*. Brighton: Harvester Wheatsheaf.

Cockerham, G.B. and Cockerham, W.C., 2010. *Health and globalization*. Cambridge: Polity.

Collier, P., 2007. *The bottom billion*. Oxford: Oxford University Press.

Collin, J., Lee, K., and Bissell, K., 2002. The framework convention on tobacco control: the politics of global heath governance. *Third World Quarterly*, 23 (2), 265–282.

Davidoff, F., Haynes, B., Sackett, D., and Smith, R., 1995. Evidence based medicine. *British Medical Journal*, 310 (6987), 1085–1086.

Davies, S., 2008. Securitizing infectious disease. *International Affairs*, 84 (2), 295–313.

Department of Health [DoH], 2008. *Health is global: a government strategy 2008–13*. London: HMSO.

Dodgson, R., Lee, K., and Drager, N., 2002. *Global health governance: a conceptual review*. LSHTM/WHO Discussion Paper No. 1. Available from: http://whqlibdoc.who.int/publications/2002/a85727_eng.pdf [Accessed 1 November 2011].

Dorfman, L. and Woodruff, K., 2005. More than a message: framing public health advocacy to change corporate practices. *Health Education and Behavior*, 32 (3), 320–336.

Entman, R.M., 1993. Framing: toward clarification of a fractured paradigm. *Journal of Communication*, 43 (4), 51–58.

Escobar, A., 1995. *Encountering development: the making and unmaking of the Third World*. Princeton, PA: Princeton University Press.

Escobar, A., 2004. Beyond the Third World: imperial globality, global coloniality and anti-globalisation social movements. *Third World Quarterly*, 25 (1), 207–230.

Farmer, P., 2003. *Pathologies of power: health human rights and the new war on the poor*. Berkeley, CA: University of California Press.

Fee, E. and Parry, M., 2008. Jonathan Mann, HIV/AIDS and human rights. *Journal of Public Health Policy*, 29, 54–71.

Fidler, D., 2004. Germs, governance and global public health in the wake of SARS. *Journal of Clinical Investigation*, 113 (6), 799–804.

Fidler, D., 2010. Influenza virus samples, international law and global health diplomacy. *Emerging Infectious Diseases*, 14 (1), 88–94.

Finnemore, M. and Sikkink, K., 1998. International norm dynamics and political change. *International Organization*, 52 (2), 887–917.

Fischer, F., ed. 2003. *Reframing public policy: discursive politics and deliberative practices*. Oxford: Oxford University Press.

George, A., 1979. Case studies and theory development: the method of structured, focused comparison. *In*: P. Lauren, ed. *Diplomacy: new approaches in history, theory and policy*. New York: Free Press, 43–69.

Gitlin, T., 1980. *The whole world is watching: the mass media in the making and the unmaking of the left*. Berkeley, CA: University of California Press.

Gray, C.S., 2009. *National security dilemmas: challenges and opportunities*. Washington, DC: Potomac.

Hewson, M. and Sinclair, T.J., eds. 1999. *Approaches to global governance theory.* Albany, NY: SUNY Press.

Hunt, P., 2004. The right of everyone to the enjoyment of the highest attainable standard of physical and mental health. Report of the Special Rapporteur. Geneva: Commission on Human Rights, Economic and Social Council, United Nations.

Hunt, P. and Backman, G., 2008. Health systems and the right to the highest attainable standard of health. *Health and Human Rights*, 10 (1), 81–92.

Jerit, J., 2008. Issue framing and engagement: rhetorical strategy in public policy debates. *Political Behavior*, 30 (1), 1–24.

Kamradt-Scott, A. and McInnes, C., 2012. The securitisation of pandemic influenza: framing, security and public policy. *Global Public Health*, [advance online publication]. doi: 10.1080/17441692.2012.725752

Kay, A. and Williams, O.D., eds. 2009. *Global health governance: crisis, institutions and political economy.* Basingstoke: Palgrave.

Kristiansen, I.S. and Mooney, G., eds. 2004. *Evidence-based medicine: in its place.* Abingdon: Routledge.

Labonté, R. and Gagnon, M.L., 2010. Framing health and foreign policy: lessons for global health diplomacy. *Globalization and Health*, 6, 14.

Mann, J.M., Gostin, L., Gruskin, S., Brennan, T., Lazzarini, Z., and Fineberg, H.V., 1994. Health and human rights. *Health and Human Rights*, 1 (1), 6–23.

Mann, J.M., Grodin, M.A., Gruskin, S., and Annas, G.A., eds. 1999. *Health and human rights: a reader.* New York: Routledge.

McInnes, C. and Lee, K., 2012. *Global health and international relations.* Oxford: Polity.

Mills, A., 1997. Leopard or chameleon? The changing character of international health economics. *Tropical Medicine and International Health*, 2 (10), 963–977.

Olesen, T., 2006. In the court of public opinion: transnational problem construction in the HIV/AIDS access campaign, 1998–2001. *International Sociology*, 21 (1), 5–30.

Ollila, E., 2005. Global health priorities–priorities of the wealthy? *Globalization and Health*, 1 (6). Available from: http://www.globalizationandhealth.com/content/1/1/6 [Accessed 12 January 2012].

Onuf, N., 1989. *A world of our making: rules and rule in social theory and international relations.* Columbia: University of South Carolina Press.

Rosenau, J.N., 1995. Governance in the twenty-first century. *Global Governance*, 1 (1), 13–43.

Rosenau, J.N. and Czempiel, E.-O., eds. 1992. *Governance without government: order and change in world politics.* Cambridge: Cambridge University Press.

Rosenberg, W. and Donald, A., 1995. Evidence based medicine: an approach to clinical problem solving. *British Medical Journal*, 310 (6987), 1122–1126.

Reubi, D., 2012. Making a human right to tobacco control: expert and advocacy networks, framing and the right to health. *Global Public Health*, [advance online publication]. doi:10.1080/17441692.2012.733948

Ruger, J.P., 2005. The changing role of the World Bank in global health in historical perspective. *American Journal of Public Health*, 95 (1), 60–70.

Ruggie, J., 1998. *Constructing the world polity.* London: Routledge.

Rushton, S., 2012. The global debate over HIV-related travel restrictions: framing and policy change. *Global Public Health*, [advance online publication]. doi:10.1080/17441692.2012.735249

Sachs, J., 2005. *The end of poverty: economic possibilities for our time.* New York: Penguin.

Sackett, D., Richardson, S., Rosenberg, W., and Haynes, B., 1995. *Evidence Based Medicine.* London: Churchill Livingston.

Sackett, D., Rosenberg, W., Muir Gray, J., Haynes, B., and Richardson, S., 1996. Evidence based medicine: what it is and what it isn't. *British Medical Journal*, 312 (7023), 71.

Shiffman, J., 2009. A social explanation for the rise and fall of global health issues. *Bulletin of the World Health Organization*, 87 (8), 608–613.

Shiffman, J. and Smith, S., 2007. Generation of political priority for global health initiatives: a framework and case study of maternal mortality. *The Lancet*, 370, 1370–1379.

Tonelli, M.R., 1998. The philosophical limits of evidence based medicine. *Academic medicine*, 73 (12), 1234–1240.

UNCESCR, 2000. General comment No. 4: the right to the highest attainable standard of health. Geneva: Office of the High Commissioner for Human Rights.

Williams, M.D., 2009. *NATO, security and risk management: from Kosovo to Kandahar.* Oxford: Routledge.

Williams, O.D., 2012. Access to medicines, market failure and market intervention: a tale of two regimes. *Global Public Health*, [advance online publication]. doi: 10.1080/17441692.2012.725753

Williams, O.D. and Rushton, S., 2011. Private actors in global health governance. *In*: S. Rushton and O.D. Williams, eds. *Partnerships and foundations in global health governance.* Basingstoke: Palgrave Macmillan, 1–28.

Woodling, M., Williams, O.D., and Rushton, S., 2012. New life in old frames: HIV, development and the 'AIDS plus MDGs' approach. *Global Public Health*, [advance online publication]. doi: 10.1080/17441692.2012.728238

Youde, J., 2005. The development of a counter-epistemic community: AIDS, South Africa and international regimes. *International Relations*, 19 (4), 421–439.

Youde, J., 2012. *Global health governance.* Oxford: Polity.

The securitisation of pandemic influenza: Framing, security and public policy

Adam Kamradt-Scott[a,b] and Colin McInnes[c]

[a]Centre for International Security Studies (CISS), University of Sydney, Sydney, Australia; [b]Faculty of Public Health and Policy, London School of Hygiene and Tropical Medicine (LSHTM), London, UK; [c]Department of International Politics, Centre for Health and International Relations (CHAIR), Aberystwyth University, Aberystwyth, UK

This article examines how pandemic influenza has been framed as a security issue, threatening the functioning of both state and society, and the policy responses to this framing. Pandemic influenza has long been recognised as a threat to human health. Despite this, for much of the twentieth century it was not recognised as a security threat. In the decade surrounding the new millennium, however, the disease was successfully securitised with profound implications for public policy. This article addresses the construction of pandemic influenza as a threat. Drawing on the work of the Copenhagen School, it examines how it was successfully securitised at the turn of the millennium and with what consequences for public policy.

Introduction

The practice and discipline of security has changed markedly over the past two decades. Security is no longer restricted to the narrow confines of military threats, and health issues are now regularly cited as one amongst a number of non-traditional security concerns that include the environment, energy, food and migration (Collins 2006, Booth 2007). Attention has primarily focused on health 'threats' that range from the more traditional (largely military) security concerns of biological weapons and bioterrorist attacks, to what are often described as 'naturally occurring' emerging and re-emerging infectious disease outbreaks (McInnes and Lee 2006, Kelle 2007, Davies 2008, 2010, Elbe 2009, 2010, Enemark 2009). In recent years, the health security agenda has been expanded even further, with scientific laboratories, food, agriculture and even certain non-communicable diseases, such as diabetes and obesity identified as posing 'a global threat' (Zimmet and Alberti 2006, WHO 2007, Katona et al. 2010). A persistent theme throughout this discussion to date, however, has been the threat presented by pandemic influenza.

Pandemic influenza remains feared by health practitioners, policymakers, security experts and politicians alike. In the previous century alone, three influenza pandemics in 1918, 1957 and 1968 contributed to millions of human fatalities, as well as caused widespread social and economic disruption. Even prior to the 1918 pandemic, which remains arguably one of the most devastating events in recorded human history, the impact of pandemic influenza on human populations was well documented. Although pandemic influenza has therefore been recognised as a public health hazard for centuries, it has not always been constructed as a security threat risking political, economic or social stability. Most notably during the Cold War, when the threat of superpower confrontation dominated western security thinking, pandemic influenza was not considered a security threat at all, despite calls from some for it to be recognised as such. And even when it has been successfully securitised, the cyclical nature of the epidemic has been replicated by a subsequent period of de-securitisation. Therefore, by the 1990s, despite pandemic influenza having been recognised as a public health hazard for centuries and despite past attempts at securitisation, the disease had not been institutionalised as a security issue.

This article traces how pandemic influenza has been framed as a security threat over the past two decades and the eventual success (and limitations) of this framing.[1] In doing so, the article draws its theoretical inspiration from the Copenhagen School's securitisation theory (Buzan *et al.* 1998). Buzan *et al.* describe their project as to 'explore the logic of security itself to find out what differentiates security ... from that which is merely political' (p. 5). They argue (p. 26) that successfully labelling an issue as 'security' takes it beyond the realm of normal political discourse and allows exceptional actions to be undertaken. Crucially, '[an] issue becomes a security issue ... not necessarily because a real existential threat exists but because the issue is presented as a threat' (p. 24). The process by which this happens is securitisation, 'the positioning through speech acts (usually by a political leader) of a particular issue as a threat to survival, which, in turn, (with the consent of the relevant constituency) enables emergency measures and the suspension of "normal politics" in dealing with that issue' (McDonald 2008, p. 567). It is the (re)presentation of an issue as an existential threat that makes a speech act a securitising move.

At this point, two clarifications are necessary. First, for a securitising move to be made, the speech act need not use the term 'security', but rather a range of terms may be deployed, which demand action outside the norm. What is therefore important is not the term itself, but the implication from the use of this term that 'business as usual' will not suffice and extraordinary measures are required. Thus, the term 'threat' can be used in a securitising move and is indeed extensively used with regard to pandemic influenza.[2] But the term is also commonly used in a wide range of other health issues, not all of which are considered security issues. For example, discussions on tobacco, diabetes, cardio-vascular disease and obesity all frequently deploy the term 'threat', but none are considered security issues. For example the difference concerns levels of analysis: whether the threat is not simply to individual human health but to the functioning of the state and society. In the Copenhagen School's terms, the speech act must claim that an issue represents an *existential threat* to the state and society. Thus, although tobacco, diabetes, and so on, are all threats to human health, pandemic influenza is different in that it is also claimed to represent an existential threat to the state. This is where a second clarification is required. As McInnes and Lee (2005) have argued elsewhere, health issues rarely represent existential threats to the state in the way in which nuclear weapons or invasion might;

but neither do many other issues which are considered 'security' threats. Thus, the term 'existential' as used by the Copenhagen School appears to set the threshold excessively high and 'extreme' or 'exceptional' might be a more accurate description of the nature of the threat.

Much of the Copenhagen School's work concerns the *process* of securitisation, and the process of securitising pandemic influenza is the focus of this article. At the heart of the securitisation theory is a 'triology' (Stritzel 2007, p. 358, 362) of speech act: the securitising move, which, as Williams [2003, pp. 524–528] notes, may use images and other 'communicative practices' rather than or as well as words[3]; the securitising actor, who makes the speech act; and the audience, who accept or reject the securitising move. This allows us to adopt a heuristic divide between the securitising move, made by an actor who can speak with authority on the issue, and successful securitisation, which is the acceptance of the securitising move by an epistemic community (the audience) which can then take emergency action on the issue. Five points should, however, be noted at the outset. First, although the Copenhagen School has provided one of the most compelling accounts of how issues can be successfully framed as security issues, large elements of the securitisation theory remain contested (see, for example, McSweeney 1996, Hansen 2000, Williams 2003, Stritzel 2007, McDonald 2008, Ciută 2009). Of particular importance to this article is that this includes the conditions necessary for successful securitisation. In this, we follow the work of Balzacq (2005, 2011) in arguing that context and material events play a role in the securitising process. Second, and following this latter point, not all securitising moves are successful. There was therefore no guarantee that calls for pandemic influenza to be treated as a security threat meriting emergency actions would create a pathway for policy responses. Third, and related to this, securitisation is not a binary condition whereby an issue is either securitised or not, but a continuum where different elements of the audience may hold different positions, and along which a consensus may shift over time.[4] Fourth, although the securitising act and its acceptance may be usefully considered as distinct for heuristic purposes here, this distinction is not always clear cut, especially if the acceptance by an epistemic community at one level (e.g. within a state or an organisation) then becomes a securitising move for another level (e.g. internationally, see McInnes and Rushton, 2012). Finally, the Copenhagen School is a normative project, which emphasises that securitisation is not necessarily a desirable state given the negative consequences involved, including suspension of basic rights and freedoms; rather, they promote ideas of 'de-securitisation'. This theoretical move allows us to introduce the idea that securitisation may not always be a linear event whereby once an issue has been securitised it will remain so. However, given the fact that the process is largely contingent upon audience acceptance and recognition, de-securitisation can also occur. As a result, the process may be understood as a cyclical event, one where a process of re-validation must take place in order for an issue to remain securitised.

The historicisation of pandemic influenza as a security threat

The framing of pandemic influenza as a security threat is not a recent phenomenon. Indeed, due to the persistent nature of the hazard, the perceived 'threat' arising from pandemic influenza has become embedded to such an extent that 'it is implicitly assumed that when we talk about this issue we are by definition in the area of urgency' (Buzan *et al.* 1998, p. 28). Much of this can be attributed to the fact that influenza epidemics and pandemics have been a persistent feature of recorded human existence for the better part of a thousand years (Kamradt-Scott 2012). Throughout the majority of those centuries, the etiological agent responsible (a virus from the Orthomyxoviridae family) remained unknown; yet, the symptoms of the disease were well recognised, so much so that the impact of influenza epidemics upon civilian populations has been extensively documented. Added to this, the frequency with which influenza pandemics have occurred (most notably in the years 1557–1580, 1781–1782, 1830–1833, 1889–1892, 1918–1919, 1957, 1968 and 2009) broadly suggests that such events can be expected to occur approximately every 40 to 50 years. As a result of such frequency, since the late eighteenth century, most generations have experienced an influenza pandemic at some point throughout their lives and have most certainly been affected by seasonal variants.

The threat of pandemic influenza to the state has also manifested itself in much more explicit security terms as well. Governments have paid close attention to the impact of influenza epidemics and pandemics on military readiness since at least 1782 (Hirsch 1883, Parsons 1891) while the influenza pandemic of 1918 was erroneously named the 'Spanish Flu' because of fears over signalling military weakness (Beveridge, 1977, 42; Potter 1991). In this, and crucially for our purposes, the 1918 Spanish Flu pandemic has become a watershed event in the historicisation of pandemic influenza as an existential threat and the establishment of a contemporary narrative of the disease as a security concern (see, for example, Osterholm 2005, Enemark 2009, Koblentz 2009). In many ways, this is not particularly surprising given the magnitude of human fatalities throughout the 1918 influenza pandemic. In the aftermath of the 1918 Spanish Flu pandemic, however, influenza also attracted the reputation as a 'war disease' (Francis 1947, p. 10). Arriving as it did at the end of the First World War, the pandemic 'irrevocably linked those two catastrophes. It demonstrated that virulent influenza may be more devastating of human life than war itself' (Francis 1958, p. 85). It was on the basis of this widespread concern that when the Second World War broke out, the US Army established a special research and development division for the creation and trial of an effective vaccine (Francis 1947). By 1944, medical professionals were arguing that 'pure and applied science' was 'fundamentally related to national security and well-being' to counter the hazard posed by influenza and other air-borne diseases (Mudd 1944, p. 445). In 1946, the interim committee charged with overseeing the creation of a new universal health organisation – the World Health Organization (WHO) – was directed to immediately create a new influenza research and surveillance centre based in London (Payne 1953). Over time, as further research centres and laboratories joined the WHO's efforts, a new global influenza surveillance network was created – a network that currently comprises over 135 public and private research institutions based in over 105 countries around the world (WHO 2011). Moreover, the risk that the world may experience a repeat of the 1918 pandemic has been periodically used as justification for free mass vaccination campaigns, such as the 1976 Swine Flu Campaign in the US (Kavet 1977, Pyhälä 1980), and the suspension of normal pharmaceutical regulatory practices such as the distribution (without prescription) of antiviral medications throughout the UK in 2009 (UK Government 2009, Elbe 2011).

These various developments have consolidated the historicisation of pandemic influenza as a security threat. Even by the 1950s, medical professionals had explicitly adopted security-related terminology such as 'threat' to describe the danger posed by pandemic influenza (Nelson 1958). Over the next three decades, concerns about the disease were overshadowed by more conventional security concerns related to the Cold War; nevertheless, periodic references to the 'threat' of pandemic influenza continued to appear and, as might be expected, were particularly intense following the influenza pandemics of 1957 and 1968. Frequently in these accounts, the 1918 pandemic was used to illustrate the wider societal (catastrophic) consequences of influenza pandemics, usually in an attempt to heighten political interest in, and argue for, increased resources for surveillance and/or vaccination programmes (Pyhälä 1980) or simply to elevate awareness and general concern (Walters 1978). These attempts to portray the disease as an 'existential threat' had limited impact in light of the threat posed by nuclear annihilation, and may be considered unsuccessful securitisations.

By the early 1990s, however, with the nuclear threat receding and the 'clear and present danger' of global war apparently consigned to the dustbin of history, governments began to grapple with new 'non-traditional' security threats. This changing context produced a permissive atmosphere so much so that towards the end of the decade emerging and re-emerging infectious diseases (ERIDs), including pandemic influenza, could begin to be discussed as *both* public health hazards *and* security risks (Garrett 1994, Glezen, 1996, Gensheimer *et al.* 1999, McInnes and Lee 2006). The significance of this heightened awareness, however, should not be overstated: when in 1997 a new strain of H5N1 influenza, that killed six out of 18 people infected, appeared in Hong Kong, the international community was ill prepared to respond, and it was only with this event that a new cycle of securitisation began that took almost a decade to successfully complete. Nevertheless, by the end of the millennium, two narratives had become well established: the historicisation of pandemic influenza as a security threat, dating back to the 1918 Spanish Flu pandemic; and the narrative of new security risks.

Securitising pandemic influenza: actors and context

Human agency is a critical factor within any framing activity, including that of securitisation. But it is only one side of the coin. As Williams (2003, 514) has observed, the process of securitisation is 'structured by the differential capacity of actors to make socially effective claims about threats, by the forms in which these claims can be made in order to be recognised and accepted as convincing by the relevant audience, and by the empirical factors or situations to which these actors can make reference'. Similarly Balzacq (2005, 2011) has argued that context plays a role in successful securitising moves. Therefore, although human agency through the speech act is integral to the process of framing, and in endorsing (or not) the frames being produced, equally important is the need for the frames to be based on an accepted empirically valid reality or within a suitable context.

Nevertheless, actors remain crucial to the securitisation of pandemic influenza in framing the disease as an existential threat requiring emergency action. The implication of this is that pandemic influenza is not *naturally* a security threat but rather needs to be *constructed* as such. DeLacy (1993, pp. 63–64) has argued, for

Table 1. Google Scholar search results for articles with 'pandemic influenza' and with 'security' or 'threat' included in title between 1950 and 2009 (as of 1 September 2011).

Year(s)	No. of articles with 'pandemic influenza' only included in title	No. of articles with 'pandemic influenza' and 'security' or 'threat' in title
1950–1959	4	0
1960–1969	3	0
1970–1979	25	0
1980–1989	21	0
1990–1999	66	3
2000–2009	1,750	67

instance, that in the eighteenth century influenza was not understood as posing a direct threat to social stability but rather 'doctors and patients alike knew that it was persuasive but rarely fatal... For most people it was a nuisance, not a disaster'. The 1918 influenza pandemic, however, provided the context for subsequent generations of health practitioners and academics, often using economic modelling and statistical studies, to begin framing influenza as a security threat through not simply its effect on morbidity and mortality, but through its potential effects on economic and social stability. This framing was a slow process that accelerated around the turn of the millennium with events, such as the 1997 H5N1 outbreak, the 2003 SARS outbreak, the global dissemination of the H5N1 influenza virus and the 2009 influenza pandemic providing a context of renewed urgency (see Tables 1, 2 and 3). But what was also vital was the mix and extent of actors engaging in securitising speech acts which, when combined with the positions of authority they maintained, helped guarantee that the threat claims were widely accepted. As Marston and Watts (2003) have observed, 'Formal hierarchies in policy communities are... potentially important factors in framing policy problems and solutions. Ministerial advisers, senior public servants, and other 'insiders' or 'policy elites' have greater access and authority in decision-making processes than members of the public or service users' (p. 145). Moreover, the agents engaging in these securitising moves extended from individuals to professional groups to global institutions. At the individual level, actors engaging in securitising moves have ranged from prominent health and medical practitioners, such as Michael T. Osterholm, Kathleen F. Genshimer and Anthony S. Fauci, to academics, such as Lawrence Gostin, David P. Fidler, Stefan Elbe, Andrew T.

Table 2. Google Scholar search results for articles with 'pandemic influenza' and with 'security' or 'threat' between 1990 and 2011 (as of 1 September 2011).

Year(s)	No. of articles with 'pandemic influenza' only included in title	No. of articles with 'pandemic influenza' and 'security' or 'threat' in title	No. of articles with 'pandemic influenza' and 'security' or 'threat' anywhere in article
1990–1996	33	0	56
1997–2003	137	6	363
2004–2008	1,070	54	3,600*
2009–2011	2,320	17	3,580

* = approximately.

Table 3. *New York Times* search results for articles on pandemic and avian influenza, and with articles that include 'security' or 'threat' between 1990 and 2011 (as of 1 September 2011).

Year(s)	No. of articles on 'pandemic influenza'	No. of articles on 'avian influenza'	No. of articles on 'pandemic influenza' or 'avian influenza' and 'security' or 'threat' anywhere in article
1990–1996	1	0	1
1997–2003	0	36	2
2004–2008	32	455	13
2009–2011	15	27	1

Price-Smith and Christian Enemark (Koblentz 2010), through to senior policymakers and politicians, such as former Democratic Senator and now US President Barack Obama (see Obama and Lugar 2005). Similarly, journalists such as Laurie Garrett, who serves as an advisor to the US Council of Foreign Relations and has addressed US Senate Committees on the 'threat' of pandemic influenza, further reinforced the securitisation framing (Garrett 2005a, 2005b). The threatening nature of pandemic influenza has been repeatedly emphasised by the medical profession (Vance 2011).

In addition, various armed forces have been complicit in framing pandemic influenza as a security threat. In 1997, for example, the US Department of Defense established a military-operated Global Laboratory-based Influenza Surveillance Programme (Owens *et al.* 2009), partly in response to an outbreak of influenza on a US navy vessel in 1996 that affected approximately 42% of the 600-person crew (95% of whom had received influenza vaccinations) (Amelio *et al.* 2002). The core function of this programme, which was further expanded upon in 1998 with the creation of the Global Emerging Infections Surveillance and Response System (DoD-GEIS), is to conduct surveillance for influenza-like illnesses (Sueker *et al.* 2010). Adding even further weight to these claims have been several very prominent institutions, the most notable being the WHO, which asserted that pandemic influenza existed as 'the most feared security threat' (WHO 2007, p. 45); the US National Intelligence Council that identified pandemic influenza as one of the 'most dangerous' threats to US national interests' (NIC 2000, p. 6); and the United Nations that – at the request of member states – established an entirely new supra-institutional office to respond to the pandemic influenza threat.

The intent behind these actions has, in many instances, been deliberate. For example, Andrew Cassels, WHO Director of Strategy for the Office of the Director-General, recently commented in relation to the WHO that:

> The security and economic arguments have gone hand in hand. First of all it was about bringing HIV/AIDS to the forefront of the agenda, but then it expanded to include deliberate release. In part though, it has also been about securing political and financial support for the organisation. Bringing health issues into the security domain has been a fairly deliberate strategy-one that has been criticised by some Member States admittedly, but one that has probably been inevitable. (Interview 22, March 2010)

At the same time, other actors suggest that it has been less about strategic framing *per se*, but rather about using the most appropriate language to communicate effectively with stakeholders, as David Nabarro, Executive Director of UNSIC, recalled:

> We have found that when we're talking to a larger group of stakeholders we have to modify our language a lot…and I am very, very keen that we take a broader disciplinary, or multi-disciplinary approach to dealing with pandemic influenza. Sometimes, in this context, we have to modify not just the title that we use with terminology like 'health security', but also the nature of our discourse. (Interview 27, October 2010)

Importantly, however, although such an approach is more nuanced, by intentionally re-moulding the language to suit a particular audience, these actors are still engaging in a framing exercise. Moreover, the objective – namely, to highlight a particular issue that requires resources and/or emergency measures – frequently remains the same, irrespective of whether the framing exercise was overt or not. As Ann Moen, Associate Director for Extramural Program, Influenza Division, US Centers for Disease Control and Prevention, summarised, 'Any chance to get funding and resources that also spotlights flu is good for our efforts to build capacity for surveillance, laboratory and pandemic preparedness globally' (Interview 20, October 2010).

Collectively, the securitising speech acts by this wide range of actors and the frequency with which they have been deployed since 1997 have had a demonstrable impact, revealing a measure of audience acceptance. Evidence of this can be found in three key areas. First, according to UNSIC, most governments have adhered to the advice of the WHO and now developed national pandemic preparedness plans (UNSIC and World Bank 2010). Second, the majority of countries that possessed the financial means to do so entered into advance purchase agreements worth billions of dollars with pharmaceutical manufacturers to secure access to antiviral medications and influenza vaccines to protect their respective populations (Mounier-Jack et al. 2007). Third, between 2005 and 2009, governments pledged US$4.3 billion towards strengthening global pandemic preparedness and by 2010 some US$2.7 billion of this had already been disbursed (UNSIC and World Bank 2010). In short, the securitisation of pandemic influenza had a remarkable effect, mobilising considerable resources and prompting extensive planning and preparation, including the passage of new regulations and laws that, importantly, justify and codify a range of emergency measures that extend from social distancing practices to law enforcement and quarantine. More recently, security concerns relating to scientific experiments involving genetic manipulation of the H5N1 avian influenza virus into an airborne strain have resulted in information being (voluntarily, but very reluctantly) withheld from publication, and a self-imposed moratorium on further research while the international community debates the moral and security concerns relating to 'dual-use' influenza research (WHO 2012). In other words, securitising pandemic influenza appeared to create a pathway for emergency responses to be undertaken outside the normal planning realm, and has contributed, and is contributing, to small but significant social changes in contemporary society.

To what extent, however, was this range of actions the product of labelling pandemic influenza a security issue, as opposed to a public health policy response to an imminent emergency? Methodologically, of course, addressing a counter-factual – what would have been different if the securitising move had not been successful – is problematic (Fearon, 1991). Nevertheless, the work done by framing the issue as a security threat is central to the broader project of which this case study is part (see McInnes and others, this issue). There are three reasons to suspect that securitisation performed a major role in generating these policy responses. Although some of these might appear as much correlations as causations, taken together we believe they represent substantial evidence that framing pandemic influenza as a security threat meant that the policy response was different in scale and character to that of a public health response. First, the synchronicity between the securitising move and these emergency actions is significant. Although the potential for pandemic influenza to result in large numbers of human fatalities had been identified prior to securitisation, emergency actions in terms of planning and advance purchasing of vaccines only occurred once the securitising process had been undertaken. And, although the response was clearly affected by health events (such as SARS and the 2005 H5N1 outbreak), the fact that these were framed as security issues rather than solely public health was, we believe, significant and in no small part explains the difference in response with the 1957 and 1968 outbreaks of pandemic influenza when the disease was not successfully securitised. Second, the form of the response differed from one solely motivated by public health concerns. For example, a public health response would have prioritised the stockpiling of anti-virals and vaccines for use where needed. This would have been motivated both by the ethical priorities of health professionals (addressing need and reducing harm) and epidemiology (to prevent the further spread of the disease). Moreover, global planning would have been prioritised – at least to some extent – to ensure a coherent response, especially given the dominant narrative of health as a global concern. However, what emerged were a series of national agreements to advance purchase drugs and national plans for pandemic preparedness only loosely coordinated at the global level. In other words, national security was prioritised over global public health. Third, interviews conducted as part of this project supported the view that security had been an important lever in motivating emergency action by governments.

Pandemic influenza securitised: the impact on public policy

The 1997 H5N1 influenza outbreak in Hong Kong marked the beginning of a new cycle in the securitisation of pandemic influenza. As the lead technical agency charged with coordinating international health work, the WHO was caught unprepared at the time of the outbreak, having reduced the number of influenza-dedicated staff in the WHO headquarters in Geneva, Switzerland, reportedly to just one individual (Kamradt-Scott 2012). However, due to a concurrent process that had been initiated in 1995 to revise the International Health Regulations (IHR) and the WHO's outbreak response policies, the organisation was able to rapidly assemble a Pandemic Task Force and, following a formal request from the Hong Kong administration, send an investigative team to assist health authorities contain the outbreak (Snacken et al. 1998). Although controversial at the time, the decision by Hong Kong's then health minister, Dr. Margaret Chan, to eliminate the territory's entire poultry population contained the outbreak and no further cases of human or avian H5N1 cases were recorded.

The 1997 outbreak spurred considerable activity in pandemic planning and preparation. In 1999, for example, the WHO published its first official guidance document in which the organisation outlined a number of pandemic 'phases' and articulated a clear need for all countries to develop national pandemic plans and strengthen their response capacities against the 'pandemic threat' (WHO 1999).

Using Vuori's (2008) classification, this appears to be a 'claim speech act' in that it attempted to raise an issue on decision makers' agendas. With such claims 'the speaker has to present or to have proof for the truth of his/her claim and it should not be obvious to both the speaker and the hearer that the hearer knows the truth of the claim already' (Vuori 2008, p. 77). Events such as the 2001 anthrax letter attacks in the US further reinforced the need to develop health security-related contingency plans (Gensheimer *et al.* 2003); and in the immediate years that followed, governments, particularly of Western populations, launched a raft of initiatives aimed at developing and testing national pandemic influenza contingency measures. Plans were developed using scenarios supported by epidemic modelling and clinical attack rates, often based on the 1918 pandemic, to predict the extent of projected human morbidity and mortality (Tam 1999). Economic studies examining potential impacts to national productivity, and social and economic functioning were similarly used to evaluate mitigation strategies (such as vaccination programmes), to inform policy and justify the need for further pandemic planning (Meltzer *et al.* 1999, Gust *et al.* 2001). These modelling exercises and scenarios, many of which were government-initiated or commissioned by state-sponsored research funding, frequently emphasised the catastrophic consequences of a widespread pandemic. In so doing, they further bolstered the case that pandemic influenza not only presented an immediate threat to human well-being but also directly threatened the state via massive social and economic disruption.

Despite these indications that pandemic influenza had been securitised – in that governments were taking emergency actions in response to securitising claims – ultimately, between 1997 and 2003, the extent of the response was limited. Indeed, even though a wide range of actors, including government officials, health practitioners, policymakers, representatives of international and regional organisations and scholars, had been fully complicit in framing pandemic influenza as a security threat – and that decision makers appeared to have been successfully persuaded of this, resulting in the authorisation of new pandemic plans – ultimately, practical measures in strengthening international response capabilities (such as enhancing overall global vaccine production capacity) were comparatively few. Thus, although pandemic influenza had been securitised, the priority given to it appeared low in comparison with other threats. This supports the idea articulated earlier that securitisation is not a binary condition but a continuum along which consensus over the issue and over the necessity for emergency action may vary. At this time, pandemic influenza clearly appeared to be only part way along the continuum to full securitisation.

In November 2003, confirmation that a new, highly virulent strain of H5N1 avian influenza had begun infecting humans and was spreading progressively throughout Asia provided the material event allowing pandemic influenza to move further along this continuum to full securitisation. Importantly, however, this occurred within the context of heightened security anxieties and of increased global sensitivities over infectious disease. The 11 September 2001 terrorist attacks on New York and Washington, the war with Afghanistan and then, in March 2003, the invasion of Iraq following concerns over its development of weapons of mass destruction, all provided a context of heightened anxiety over security. Contemporaneous with the invasion of Iraq, a novel pathogen began spreading internationally from Hong Kong. The subsequent global dissemination of the SARS-associated coronavirus between

March and July 2003 proved a distressing reminder of the human, economic and social consequences that accompanied disease outbreaks in a highly interconnected world. The entire global outbreak resulted in just over 8000 cases and approximately 800 fatalities, and yet the economic damage to the Asia-Pacific region alone from SARS was estimated at over US$30 billion (WHO 2007). To many health practitioners and policymakers SARS was seen as a 'wake-up call' (Campbell 2004, p. 5), and the outbreak generated significant political commitment not only to conclude revising the IHRs but also to ensure greater international cooperation in tackling disease threats (Kamradt-Scott 2010). Within a few months of SARS having been successfully contained, however, several small outbreaks of the H5N1 avian influenza virus (which later became commonly referred to as 'Bird Flu') were recorded in Southeast Asia. Throughout 2004, the number of outbreaks increased, and despite several containment exercises targeting domestic bird populations, several countries that had never recorded outbreaks began reporting new human cases of H5N1 (Webster and Govorkova 2006). As a result, new pressure was applied to politicians, both domestically and internationally, to better respond to what was clearly being portrayed as an emerging threat.

By 2005, persuaded by the growing threat of H5N1 influenza (Obama and Lugar 2005), governments the world over implemented a range of new pandemic planning and preparation activities. Moreover, government officials were so persuaded by the threat of pandemic influenza that the need for comprehensive pandemic planning was presented to citizens as self-evident (Stephenson and Jamieson 2009). At the urging of several Southeast Asian countries, the Secretary-General of the United Nations established a new department – the United Nations System Influenza Coordinator, or UNSIC – to coordinate the multiple UN agencies engaged in activities related to preventing avian influenza. The creation of this supra-organisational entity coincided with the founding of the International Partnership on Avian and Pandemic Influenza by US President George W. Bush and the allocation of significant US government funds for strengthening international surveillance, detection and response (Osterholm 2007). Around the world, individual governments sought to strengthen their own domestic response capacity by implementing H5N1 testing of domestic poultry and agreeing to contracts worth billions of dollars with pharmaceutical manufacturers to purchase large quantities of antiviral medications and influenza vaccines (Mounier-Jack et al. 2007, Lam 2008). Intergovernmental organisations, such as the WHO, the Association of Southeast Asian Nations (ASEAN) and the Asia-Pacific Economic Cooperation (APEC) received new injections of financial support from their respective member states to enhance pandemic influenza preparedness and response capabilities. Various local, national, regional and international plans were developed, and in a number of instances exercised. Consultation meetings were convened; new laws and regulations were passed. In short, the international community entered what may be described as pandemic overdrive, pledging, between 2005 and 2009, approximately US$4.3 billion to enhance global pandemic preparedness (UNSIC and World Bank 2010).

In April 2009, the hyperactivity that accompanied the global spread of H5N1 influenza initially seemed to have been validated following the announcement that yet another new strain of H1N1 influenza had successfully begun to infect humans. Within a matter of weeks, the virus that had originally emerged in Mexico had been detected in multiple countries around the world. As the WHO moved to declare a full-scale pandemic, the governments of affected countries executed their respective pandemic plans and initiated various emergency measures. These ranged from thermal screening at airports, quarantine and isolation of suspected and confirmed cases, cancellation of mass gatherings, school and child care centre closures and the procurement of mass quantities of antiviral medications and influenza vaccines. In some instances, governments willingly contravened sound scientific advice by implementing measures, such as quarantining all Mexican citizens within their borders, banning the import of all live pigs and pork products and, in the particular case of Egypt, slaughtering the country's entire pig population due to initial depictions of the virus as 'Swine Flu' (Hodge 2010, Katz and Fischer 2010), ostensibly to demonstrate their commitment to protecting populations from infection. Indeed, throughout all this activity, prime ministers, presidents, senior government officials, health practitioners and policymakers were repeatedly observed emphasising the threat the influenza pandemic presented, as well as justifying the various measures they were taking to protect public health.

Conclusion

Unlike the securitisation of HIV/AIDS that others have argued is a recent phenomenon (Elbe 2006, McInnes and Rushton 2012), the framing of pandemic influenza as a threat to national and international security has been an extensive one, extending over decades as opposed to years. Clearly, the 1918 influenza pandemic has been the key milestone in this framing exercise; but there is little question that the most intensive phase of this process began in the mid-1990s and came to a peak around 2005. This is not to suggest, however, that the process of framing this disease as a security threat has always been successful. Despite the numerous examples of medical professionals in the 1950s using security-related terminology to describe the hazard posed by influenza, and an acute awareness of the impact that the disease could have on the physical, economic, and social stability of societies, when confronted with the threat of nuclear annihilation brought on by the Cold War governments – perhaps understandably – accorded less attention to the threat of pandemic influenza. By the late 1990s, however, the situation had changed once again, and the disease rapidly became widely accepted as a security threat through a blending of real-world events combined with the strategic framing of the disease by socially legitimate agents. In this regard, human agency, while still integral to the process, has not been as significant in the context of framing pandemic influenza as a security threat as it has apparently been in securitising other infectious diseases, such as HIV/AIDS. Indeed, had it not been for the fact that actors sought to augment their framing attempts by drawing on economic projections and epidemiological studies of the potential catastrophic failure of society, it is uncertain whether the framing of pandemic influenza as a security threat would have been as successful as it appears to have been. The effect of framing pandemic influenza as a threat to national and international security has, however, been profound both in terms of measures undertaken and the global spread of responses. Most states, as well as key international institutions, have reacted to the construction of pandemic influenza as a threat by establishing emergency planning measures, which take responses to the disease outside the realm of 'normal politics'. In this respect, the successful framing of the disease as a security issue opened up a pathway for exceptional responses.

What is also apparent is that framing of the disease in terms of security drew additional attention to the threat from policymakers (compared to, for example, the previous pandemics of 1957 and 1968), and produced a policy response geared to national protection. The latter is significant given the successful move over the past two decades to reconstruct health as global-that global responses were required to meet global threats such as pandemic influenza. What is apparent here, however, is that preparedness, planning and policies were driven by national priorities and not the need for a coherent global public health response.

Acknowledgements

This research has been made possible through funding from the European Research Council under the European Community's Seventh Framework Programme – Ideas Grant 230489 GHG. All views expressed remain those of the authors.

Notes

1. This article draws on a range of elite interviews conducted in Geneva, London and Singapore between 2010 and 2011. For reasons of confidentiality, agreed upon with interview subjects, these are generally not cited in the text. We would also like to thank the anonymous reviewers for their comments on and suggestions for this article.
2. One implication of this is that the use of the word 'security' is not necessary in the speech act. Indeed, with pandemic influenza, the operational term appears to have been 'threat'.
3. In this context, it is interesting to examine David Campbell's work on the 'visual economy' of HIV/AIDS (Campbell 2008).
4. The issue of partial securitisation is discussed at length in McInnes and Rushton, 2012.

References

Amelio, R., Biselli, R., Cali, G., and Peragallo, M., 2002. Vaccination policies in the military: an insight on influenza. *Vaccine*, 20 (Suppl. 5), B36–B39.

Balzacq, T., 2005. The three faces of securitization: political agency, audience and context. *European journal of international relations*, 11 (2), 171–201.

Balzacq, T., 2011. A theory of securitization: origins, core assumptions, and variants. *In*: T. Balzacq, ed. *Securitization theory: how security problems emerge and dissolve*. Abingdon, UK: Routledge.

Beveridge, W., 1977. *Influenza: the last great plague*. London: Heinemann.

Booth, K., 2007. *Theory of world security*. Cambridge: Cambridge University Press.

Buzan, B., Waever, O., and de Wilde, J., 1998. *Security: a new framework for analysis*. Boulder, CO: Lynne Rienner.

Campbell, A. 2004. *The SARS commission interim report: SARS and public health in Ontario*. Ontario, Canada: The Ministry of Health and Long-Term Care. Available from: http://www. health.gov.on.ca/english/public/pub/ministry_reports/campbell04/campbell04.pdf [Accessed 6 Sept 2011].

Campbell, D. 2008. The visual economy of HIV/AIDS: a report for the AIDS, security and conflict initiative. Available from: www.david-campbell.org/wp-content/documents/Visual_ Economy_of_HIV_AIDS.pdf [Accessed 6 Aug 2012].

Ciută, F., 2009. Security and the problem of context: a hermeneutical critique of securitisation theory. *Review of international studies*, 35 (2), 301–326.

Collins, A., ed. 2006. *Contemporary security studies*. Oxford: Oxford University Press.

Davies, S., 2008. Securitizing infectious disease. *International affairs*, 84 (2), 295–313.

Davies, S., 2010. *Global politics of health*. Oxford: Polity.

DeLacy, M., 1993. Influenza research and the medical profession in eighteenth-century Britain. *Albion: a quarterly journal concerned with British studies*, 25 (1), 37–66.

Elbe, S., 2006. Should HIV/AIDS be securitised? The ethical dilemmas of linking HIV/AIDS and security. *International studies quarterly*, 50 (1), 119–144.

Elbe, S., 2009. *Virus alert: security, governmentality and the AIDS pandemic*. New York: Columbia University Press.

Elbe, S., 2010. *Security and global health: toward the medicalization of insecurity*. Cambridge: Polity.

Elbe, S., 2011. Pandemics on the radar screen: health security, infectious disease and the medicalisation of insecurity. *Political studies*, 59 (4), 848–866.

Enemark, C., 2009. Is pandemic flu a security threat? *Survival*, 51 (1), 191–214.

Fearon, J., 1991. Counterfactuals and hypothesis testing in political science. *World politics*, 43 (2), 169–195.

Francis, T., Jr. 1947. A consideration of vaccination against influenza. *The Milbank memorial fund quarterly*, 25 (1), 5–20.

Francis, T., Jr. 1958. *Influenza. Preventive Medicine in World War II, vol. IV.* Washington, DC: US Government Printing Office. Available from: http://history.amedd.army.mil/booksdocs/wwii/PM4/CH04.Influenza.htm [Accessed 29 Mar 2012].

Garrett, L., 1994. *The coming plague: newly emergent diseases in a world out of balance*. New York: Farrar, Straus and Giroux.

Garrett, L., 2005a. The next pandemic? *Foreign affairs*, 84 (4), 3–23.

Garrett, L. 2005b. Responding to the threat of global, virulent influenza. Written testimony before the United States Senate Committee on Foreign Relations, 9 November 2005. Available from: http://foreign.senate.gov/imo/media/doc/GarrettTestimony051109.pdf [Accessed 5 Sept 2011].

Gensheimer, K.F., Fukuda, K., Brammer, L., Cox, N., Patriarca, P.A., and Strikas, R.A. 1999. Preparing for pandemic influenza: the need for enhanced surveillance. *Emerging infectious diseases*, 5 (2). Available from: http://www.cdc.gov/ncidod/eid/vol5no2/gensheimer.htm [Accessed 30 Aug 2011].

Gensheimer, K.F., Meltzer, M.I., Postema, A.S., and Fukuda, K., 2003. Influenza pandemic preparedness. *Emerging infectious diseases*, 9 (12), 1645–1648.

Glezen, W.P., 1996. Emerging infections: pandemic influenza. *Epidemiologic reviews*, 18 (1), 64–75.

Gust, I.D., Hampson, A.W., and Lavanchy, D., 2001. Planning for the next pandemic of influenza. *Reviews in medical virology*, 11 (1), 59–70.

Hansen, L., 2000. The little mermaid's silent security dilemma and the absence of gender in the Copenhagen school. *Millennium: journal of international studies*, 29 (2), 285–306.

Hirsch, A., 1883. *Handbook of geographical and historical pathology: volume 1 – acute infective diseases*. London: New Sydenham Society.

Hodge, J., 2010. Global legal triage in response to the 2009 H1N1 outbreak. *Minnesota journal of law, science & technology*, 11 (2), 599–628.

Kamradt-Scott, A., 2010. The WHO secretariat, norm entrepreneurship, and global disease outbreak control. *Journal of international organizations studies*, 1 (1), 72–89.

Kamradt-Scott, A., 2012. Changing perceptions of pandemic influenza and public health responses. *American journal of public health policy*, 102 (1), 90–98.

Katona, P., Sullivan, J., and Intrilligator, M., eds. 2010. *Global biosecurity: threats and responses*. London: Routledge.

Katz, R. and Fischer, J., 2010. The revised international health regulations: a framework for global pandemic response. *Global health governance*, 3 (2), 1–18.

Kavet, J., 1977. A perspective on the significance of pandemic influenza. *American journal of public health*, 67 (11), 1063–1070.

Kelle, A., 2007. Securitization of international public health. *Global governance*, 13, 217–235.

Koblentz, G.D. 2009. The threat of pandemic influenza: why today is not 1918. *World medical & health policy*, 1 (1), Article 9, doi: 10.2202/1944-2858.1007/.

Koblentz, G.D., 2010. Biosecurity reconsidered: calibrating biological threats and responses. *International security*, 34 (4), 96–132.

Lam, P.Y., 2008. Avian influenza and pandemic influenza preparedness in Hong Kong. *Annals academy of medicine Singapore*, 37 (6), 489–496.

Marston, G. and Watts, R., 2003. Tampering with the evidence: a critical appraisal of evidence-based policy-making. *The drawing board: an Australian review of public affairs*, 3 (3), 143–163.

McDonald, M., 2008. Securitization and the construction of security. *European journal of international relations*, 14 (4), 563–587.

McInnes, C. and Lee, K., 2005. Health and security. *Tiddsskriftet Politik*, 8 (1), 33–44.

McInnes, C. and Lee, K., 2006. Health, security and foreign policy. *Review of international studies*, 32 (1), 5–23.

McInnes, C. and Rushton, S. 2012. HIV/AIDS and securitization theory. *European journal of international relations*. Online first doi:10.1177/1354066111425258.

McSweeney, B., 1996. Identity and security: Buzan and the Copenhagen School. *Review of international studies*, 22 (1), 81–93.

Meltzer, M.I., Cox, N., and Fukuda, K., 1999. The economic impact of pandemic influenza in the United States: priorities for intervention. *Emerging infectious diseases*, 5 (5), 669–671.

Mounier-Jack, S., Jas, R., and Coker, R., 2007. Progress and shortcomings in European national strategic plans for pandemic influenza. *Bulletin of the World Health Organization*, 85 (12), 923–929.

Mudd, S., 1944. Air-borne infections. *British medical journal*, 2 (4369), 444–445.

NIC (National Intelligence Council), 2000. Global infectious disease threats and its implications for the United States. National Intelligence Estimate NIE 99-17D. Available from: http://www.dni.gov/nic/special_globalinfectious.html [Accessed 5 Sept 2011].

Nelson, A.J., 1958. Evaluation of Asian influenza vaccine in an industrial population. *Canadian medical association journal*, 79, 888–891.

Obama, B. and Lugar, R., 2005. Grounding a pandemic. *New York Times*, 6 June, Available from: http://www.nytimes.com/2005/06/06/opinion/06obama.html [Accessed 2 Sept 2011].

Osterholm, M.T., 2005. Preparing for the next pandemic. *New England journal of medicine*, 352 (18), 1839–1842.

Osterholm, M.T., 2007. Unprepared for a pandemic. *Foreign affairs*, 86 (2), 47–57.

Owens, A., Canas, L., Russell, K., Neville, J., Pavlin, J., MacIntosh, V., Gray, G., and Gaydos, J., 2009. Department of Defense Global Laboratory-based Influenza Surveillance: 1998–2005. *American journal of preventive medicine*, 37 (3), 235–241.

Parsons, H.F., 1891. The influenza epidemics of 1889–90 and 1891, and their distribution in England and Wales. *British medical journal*, 2 (1597), 303–308.

Payne, A.M., 1953. The influenza programme of WHO. *Bulletin of the world health organization*, 8 (5–6), 755–774.

Potter, C.W., 1991. Chronicle of influenza pandemics. *In*: R. Webster, ed. *Textbook of influenza*. London: Blackwell Science.

Pyhälä, R., 1980. Protection by a polyvalent influenza vaccine and persistence of homologous and heterologous H1 antibodies during a period of two epidemic seasons. *Journal of hygiene Cambridge*, 84 (2), 237–245.

Snacken, R., Kendal, A.P., Haaheim, L.R., and Wood, J.M., 1998. The next influenza pandemic: lessons from Hong Kong, 1997. *Emerging infectious diseases*, 5 (2), 195–203.

Stephenson, N. and Jamieson, M., 2009. Securitizing health: Australian newspaper coverage of pandemic influenza. *Sociology of health & illness*, 31 (4), 525–539.

Stritzel, H., 2007. Towards a theory of securitization: Copenhagen and beyond. *European journal of international relations*, 13 (3), 357–383.

Sueker, J., Blazes, D., Johns, M., Blair, P., Sjoberg, P., Tjaden, J., Montgomery, J., Pavlin, J., Schnabel, D., Eick, A., Tobias, S., Quintana, M., Vest, K., Burke, R., Lindler, L., Mansfield, J., Erickson, R., Russell, K., and Sanchez, J., 2010. Influenza and respiratory disease surveillance: the US military's global laboratory-based network. *Influenza and other respiratory viruses*, 4 (3), 155–161.

Tam, T., 1999. Preparing for influenza epidemics and pandemics in the new millennium. *Canadian journal of public health*, 90 (5), 293–319.

UK Government, 2009. Explanatory memorandum to the medicines for human use (miscellaneous amendments) Regulations 2009 No. 1164, the medicines for human use (prescribing) (miscellaneous amendments) Order 2009 No. 1165, the National Health Service (charges) (amendments relating to pandemic influenza) Regulations 2009 No. 1166.

Available from: http://www.legislation.gov.uk/uksi/2009/1165/pdfs0/uksiem_20091165_en. pdf [Accessed 6 Sept 2011].

UNSIC and World Bank, 2010. *Fifth global progress report 2010: a framework for sustaining momentum*. Bangkok: World Bank.

Vance, M., 2011. Disease mongering and the fear of pandemic influenza. *International journal of health services*, 41 (1), 95–115.

Vuori, J., 2008. Illocutionary logic and strands of securitization: applying the theory of securitization to the study of non-democratic political orders. *European journal of international relations*, 14 (1), 65–99.

Walters, J.H., 1978. Influenza 1918: the contemporary perspective. *Bulletin of the New York academy of medicine*, 54 (9), 855–864.

Webster, R.G. and Govorkova, E.A., 2006. H5N1 influenza – continuing evolution and spread. *New England journal of medicine*, 355 (21), 2174–2178.

WHO (World Health Organization), 1999. *Influenza pandemic plan. The role of WHO and guidelines for national and regional planning*. Geneva: WHO. Available from: http:// whqlibdoc.who.int/hq/1999/WHO_CDS_CSR_EDC_99.1.pdf [Accessed 30 Aug 2011].

WHO, 2007. *World Health Report 2007: A safer future: global public health security in the 21st century*. Geneva: WHO.

WHO, 2011. WHO global influenza surveillance network. Available from: http://www.who.int/ csr/disease/influenza/surveillance/en/index.html [Accessed 20 Sept 2011].

WHO, 2012. Technical consultation on H5N1 research issues – consensus points. Available from: http://www.who.int/influenza/human_animal_interface/consensus_points/en/index. html [Accessed 29 Mar 2012].

Williams, M.C., 2003. Words, images, enemies: securitization and international politics. *International studies quarterly*, 47 (4), 511–531.

Zimmet, P. and Alberti, K.G., 2006. Introduction: globalization and the non-communicable disease epidemic. *Obesity*, 14 (1), 1–3.

Evidence-based medicine and the governance of pandemic influenza

Adam Kamradt-Scott[a,b]

[a]Centre for International Security Studies (CISS), University of Sydney, Sydney, Australia;
[b]Faculty of Public Health and Policy, London School of Hygiene and Tropical Medicine (LSHTM), London, UK

The conventional response of governments to protect their populations against the threat of influenza has been to ensure adequate vaccine production and/or access to supplies of vaccines and antiviral medications. This focus has, in turn, shaped the global governance structures around pandemic influenza, with collective efforts centred on facilitating virus sharing, maintaining and increasing vaccine production, and ensuring access to pharmaceuticals – responses that remain unattainable for many low- and middle-income countries (LMICs) in the short to medium term. This paper argues that this emphasis on pharmacological responses reflects a particular view of biomedicine that pays inadequate attention to the weak capacity of many health systems. In more recent years, this dynamic has been further exacerbated by the influence of evidence-based medicine (EBM) that preferences certain types of biomedical knowledge and practice. This paper explores the role that EBM has played in shaping the global governance of pandemic influenza, and how it has served to reinforce and reify the authority of particular groups of actors, including policy-makers, elected officials and the medical community. The paper concludes that only by unpacking these structures and revealing the political authority in play can alternative policy responses more appropriate to LMICs be considered.

Introduction

Influenza pandemics are a regular feature of human existence, occurring periodically and usually inflicting significant human morbidity and mortality. Throughout recorded human history there is no better example of this than the 1918 influenza pandemic that killed over 40 million people worldwide. A further two pandemics in 1957 and 1968 also occurred in the twentieth century and resulted in the deaths of approximately 2 million and 1 million people, respectively. In March 2009, the first influenza pandemic of the twenty-first century began in La Gloria, Mexico, following the emergence of a novel strain of H1N1 (A) influenza. As the World Health Organization (WHO) moved to declare a 'public health emergency of international concern', governments, concerned that the pandemic may cause large numbers of human deaths, invoked their respective pandemic plans, convened emergency committees and instituted a series of public health procedures. In most instances, the measures taken by governments were logical and reasonable and adhered to the recommendations of medical advice. Further, the majority of governments' actions aligned with the global health procedures advocated by such organisations as the WHO and the United Nations System Influenza Coordinator (UNSIC) – processes that were, importantly, also informed by contemporary (bio)medical opinion that had been based on the best available evidence (WHO 2009).

Evidence-based medicine, or EBM, has been described as a 'movement', 'method', 'collaboration' and even a 'crusade' by critics and advocates (Dobbie *et al.* 2000, Kristiansen and Mooney 2004). Originally developed in Canada in the early-1990s, EBM has been progressively and extensively integrated into contemporary medical practice around the world, instructing and informing the biomedical discipline along a series of core principles. These principles, which include that decisions are based on the best available evidence, that the problem determines the nature and source of evidence to be sought, that epidemiological and biostatistical ways of thinking provide the best evidence, that conclusions are only useful if they assist in managing patients or health care decisions, and that performance should be constantly evaluated, assist adherents of EBM to categorise and stratify all modes of scientific inquiry and knowledge into distinct 'levels of evidence' (Davidoff *et al.* 1995). Within this system, systematic literature reviews that draw on randomised controlled trials (or RCTs) that assess the efficacy of therapeutic (e.g. drug-based and surgical) interventions are classified as the 'gold standard' of evidence, followed closely by meta-analyses (systematic literature reviews that use quantitative methods to summarise the results of trials). The lowest category of evidence is expert opinion (Sackett and Rosenberg 1995).

To facilitate gold standard policy-making, a range of new global networks (such as the Cochrane Collaboration) have emerged alongside second-tier academic journals that review, critique, summarise and pass comment on the published (primary source) findings of other scientific and academic studies that evaluate patient care, develop new treatment protocols and advocate statistically validated interventions to improve health outcomes. By the late 1990s, EBM had not only been integrated into the majority of contemporary medical training programmes in university-based medical schools within Organisation for Economic Co-operation and Development (OECD) countries, but it was also being widely promoted as a practice and discipline that should inform all areas of public policy (Smith 1996, Tonelli 1998). EBM epistemic communities have thus emerged and have spread worldwide, as successive generations of medical practitioners have been trained in EBM-related statistical inference and analysis. The outcome of this process has been to embed EBM as the primary mode of scientific, rational enquiry for contemporary biomedicine and clinical practice.

In this paper, I seek to unpack the existing influenza governance arrangements to identify how biomedicine and EBM in particular have come to shape (frame) the acceptable limits of pandemic influenza public policy. More specifically, in this paper I explore how influenza vaccines and antiviral medications have, and continue to be, actively promoted as the ultimate indicator of pandemic preparedness – that is, how countries prepare for, and should the need arise, how they respond to, a new, highly virulent strain of influenza – and the effect that this focus has had in downplaying the importance of other legitimate public policy responses. To contextualise these observations, the article commences with a brief historical overview of the post-war influenza governance arrangements and how they developed. The paper then examines how influenza vaccines progressively came to occupy the centre stage of pandemic preparedness policy, and how the emergence of EBM subsequently reinforced and reified vaccines, and later antivirals, through the movement's predilection for drug-based solutions. The paper then concludes by noting the impact that EBM has had in shaping (and arguably somewhat distorting) the contemporary pandemic influenza public policy and governance arrangements to the benefit of high-income countries, while downplaying other legitimate pandemic preparedness policies and knowledge that may benefit a wider proportion of the world's population.

The development of the post-war pandemic influenza governance arrangements

Following the 1918 Spanish Influenza pandemic that decimated entire communities at the end of the First World War, public perceptions regarding influenza and the danger posed by the disease perceptibly changed (Kitler *et al.* 2002). Indeed, even though seasonal epidemics of influenza had occurred with almost clockwork frequency over the previous 300 years, for a time pandemic influenza became associated with conflict, with some public health officials even viewing it as a 'war disease' (Francis 1947, p. 10). Subsequently, in the wake of the Second World War (WWII) when the decision was made in 1946 to establish a new universal health body, one of the first tasks assigned to the organisation was to develop a new programme to monitor and study influenza. The World Influenza Centre (WIC) was founded in London in 1947 to (1) plan against the recurrence of future pandemics, (2) develop control methods to limit the impact when a pandemic did appear and (3) limit as much as possible the economic impacts of influenza epidemics and pandemics (Payne 1953). In 1950, the third World Health Assembly (WHA) requested an Expert Committee on Influenza be formed to instruct the organisation's activities. The Committee, which met for the first (and only) time in 1952, comprised nine medical professionals drawn from high-income, mainly European nations and the United States. On the basis of the Committee's recommendations, the foundation of the contemporary influenza governance arrangements was laid that same year with the creation of the Global Influenza Surveillance Network (GISN).

The premise of GISN was to build an international network of influenza research laboratories that would assist the WHO provide technical support to its member states by identifying and isolating the strains of the virus currently circulating. Samples are collected by designated National Influenza Centres (NICs) and then forwarded to WHO reference laboratories (otherwise known as WHO Collaborating Centres) where the strains are isolated and categorised. The epidemiological intelligence gathered from this network is then used to inform the development of therapeutic measures such as influenza vaccines. When the network was first established in 1952, it comprised some 40 laboratories (Jensen and Hogan 1958). By 1954, the number had grown to over 50 spread throughout 42 countries, and by 1977, GISN consisted of 98 NICs throughout 70 countries (Pereira 1979). Over the years, the number of both NICs and reference laboratories has continued to increase to the extent that GISN now comprises over 135 institutions throughout 105 countries supported by a total of six WHO Collaborating Centres based in the United Kingdom, the United States, Australia, Japan and China (WHO 2011a).

Yet despite two pandemics in 1958 and 1967 and the growth of GISN, by the mid-1990s the WHO's influenza programme had been substantially reduced both in terms of scale and impact. Overall concern regarding the majority of infectious diseases had waned amongst high-income countries due to broader 'changes in health care priorities, diminished resources and the need to focus the limited available manpower and funds on the HIV/AIDS epidemic' (WHO 1994, p. 845). Influenza subsequently commanded less attention, and as such, funds for the associated WHO programme were not as abundant as what they once were. The added success of influenza vaccines in reducing high human morbidity and mortality (demonstrated by extensive clinical trials throughout the 1950s) gave added weight to reducing international financial and human resources, as influenza came to be perceived as a largely controllable disease. Indeed, instead of collective international action, throughout the latter half of the twentieth century influenza became increasingly viewed as a disease that was the responsibility of individual governments to control – ideally through vaccination campaigns, which had been validated by biomedical techniques and knowledge as the most effective means of reducing human morbidity and mortality (Hota and McGeer 2007). Noting this downturn of interest at the international level, in 1988 the then-directors of the WHO Collaborating Centres issued a statement calling for the WHO influenza programme to be 'maintained and strengthened because, by facilitating the earliest possible detection of new epidemic strains of influenza virus and recommending the use of new antigenic variants for vaccines, it provides the foundation for activities to prevent and control the disease' (WHO 1988, p. 457). The call, however, went unheeded, and while the 'threat' from 'emerging and re-emerging infectious diseases' was gaining political attention throughout the mid-1990s (Lederberg 1996), and notable virologists such as Robert Webster were warning the world was 'overdue' for another influenza pandemic (Webster 1994, Webster and Kawaoka 1994), by 1996 the number of WHO personnel overseeing the organisation's influenza work had been reduced to one staff member (Kamradt-Scott 2012).

In fact, political interest in the WHO's influenza programme only really re-emerged in 1997 following an outbreak of H5N1 avian influenza in Hong Kong that killed six out of 18 infected people (Snacken *et al.* 1999). While small in terms of overall human morbidity and mortality, the outbreak caused significant interna-tional anxiety that a new pandemic was imminent. As a result, Hong Kong's health minister, Margaret Chan, controversially ordered the destruction of the territory's entire poultry on the grounds that it was the most appropriate action to take – a decision that was reportedly based on the epidemiological evidence (Shuchman 2007). The subsequent medical consensus that emerged was that Chan's actions likely prevented a new pandemic (MacPhail 2009), but the outbreak renewed international pressure on the WHO to reinvigorate its influenza programme and the organisation immediately began developing new policy guidelines on how its member states should prepare for mitigating an influenza pandemic. The WHO's first official pandemic influenza preparedness guideline document was then released in 1999, and outlined in broad terms the steps that countries should take in developing vaccination and other control strategies, strengthening surveillance systems and ensuring access to critical supplies such as vaccines and personal protective equipment to protect their respective populations (WHO 1999).

Between 1997 and late 2003, political interest in influenza prevention and control continued to fluctuate, but following confirmation in early 2004 of widespread outbreaks of avian influenza throughout several East Asian countries, the WHO's influenza programme has remained in a perpetual state of heightened alert (WHO 2005a). Moreover, in response to the progressive spread of the H5N1 avian influenza virus and the perceived threat this disease presented to the international community (see Kamradt-Scott and McInnes this issue), by late 2005 influenza governance arrangements had expanded considerably. The creation of UNSIC, led by David Nabarro (a UK-trained medical practitioner), was joined by multiple international organisations such as the Food and Agriculture Organization (FAO), the World Bank, the International Monetary Fund (IMF) and the World Organization for Animal Health (OIE) also launching various programmes aimed at improving human and animal influenza surveillance and response. These international organisations were also joined in their efforts by regional organisations such as the Association of Southeast Asian Nations (ASEAN) and the Asia-Pacific Economic Cooperation (APEC), while at the national level many governments formed pandemic emergency planning committees. The WHO, which had commissioned a number of regional and international consultation meetings throughout 2004 and 2005, released updated pandemic preparedness documents urging member states to ramp up their efforts to prepare against the risk of another pandemic (WHO 2005b). In short, the international community went into pandemic hyper-drive.

Importantly, and as is explored in greater detail below, medical practitioners and medical knowledge have – quite understandably – been central throughout the construction and subsequent growth of the international community's post-war influenza governance arrangements. From the creation of the WHO's Expert Committee on Influenza in 1952 to the present day, medical professionals habitually retain key advisory positions ranging from the sub-national to international levels that help establish and delineate public health policy with regard to influenza prevention and control. Many would see this influence as both reasonable and appropriate, given the nature of the issues involved. Indeed, it makes rational sense to have medical experts advising on medical matters. Nonetheless, as this article seeks to draw out, medical knowledge that does not take into account broader socio-political and economic considerations can have unintended consequences not only on public policy but also on governance institutions and arrangements.

The use of biomedical and EBM techniques and knowledge in pandemic preparedness

The centrality of biomedical knowledge, techniques, processes, interventions and personnel to the control of influenza was made apparent from the inception of the WHO's influenza programme in 1947 (Kamradt-Scott forthcoming). Even so, while Pope (2003, p. 269) has observed, 'The idea that scientific research should be a component of medical knowledge was, of course, not new', following the introduction and codification of EBM practices in the mid-1990s, demand for 'evidence' in the form of results derived from RCTs and clinical trials, epidemiological modelling, and statistical analysis and inference has become even greater. As one senior WHO official recently noted:

...in the early days of EBM it was treated as 'oh bah-humbug, you don't want to do this rubbish', through to a few years ago where the students were saying 'well, why are you even teaching us about evidence, of course you've got to use it'. Evidence-based approaches had become so accepted in a relatively short period of time. (Interview 23 March 2010)

In part, this trend can be traced to broader social changes linked to the political exploitation of expert knowledge (Boswell 2009), but, as David Nabarro, the executive director of UNSIC, has observed in a recent interview, the demand that has arisen for evidence over the past 20 years is for a particular type of evidence:

Evidence is absolutely critical in the dialogue with policymakers, but it's a particular kind of evidence that's needed. You have to be able to answer particular kinds of questions. If we have a choice, says the policy maker, should we be investing in vaccination for five percent of our population, or a massive drive on hand-washing and other forms of interpersonal hygiene for, say, ninety-five percent of our population. (Interview 27 October 2010)

Further, officials within leading governance institutions like the WHO feel under pressure to incorporate EBM principles as it influences how the institutions themselves are perceived, as Tim Evans, former WHO Assistant Director-General for Information, Evidence and Research, noted:

What we've found is that it isn't a function of simply having a cluster or group of staff dedicated to a particular project, it's really the competencies of the institution as a whole, and its technical mandate, that will be increasingly judged on its ability to manage the evidence. And if we're seen not to be at least close to the cutting edge in terms of systems for assessing and evaluating evidence, then we're very legitimately open to critique. (Interview 24 March 2010)

In relation to pandemic influenza, the securitisation of the disease that occurred throughout the 1990s heightened the perceived need for governments to adopt proven and effective containment and mitigation strategies. The arrival of EBM, which emphasised that scientific data could (and should) be used to answer specific policy questions and/or problems, thereby proved especially timely, and EBM rapidly became central to understanding how governments could ensure they were more effectively prepared against the threat of pandemic influenza.

Within this context, attention predictably first turned to influenza vaccines, which since the 1950s had been actively promoted as the 'cornerstone' of effective epidemic and pandemic influenza preparedness due to extensive clinical testing validating their efficacy (Ruben 1987, Hota and McGeer 2007). Coinciding with the emergence of EBM, a number of prominent RCTs were published in the mid-1990s in respected scholarly journals, further confirming the importance of influenza vaccines (see, e.g. Nichol *et al.* 1995). At the same time, it was also widely recognised that any strategy that relied solely on influenza vaccines would be insufficient due to the time required to develop a new, pandemic-specific vaccine. A second, more reliable solution was thereby sought (and found) in the form of antiviral medications, which were to be used as a means to delay the onset of a full-scale pandemic until such time as an appropriate vaccine could be produced in sufficient quantities to launch a widespread vaccination campaign.

Intriguingly though, in contrast to the wide array of clinical evidence demonstrating the effectiveness of influenza vaccines, even by 2003 very few RCTs had been conducted to assess the efficacy of antiviral medications in the treatment of influenza (Stiver 2003). Further, many of the clinical trials that had been conducted were deemed inconclusive (Ward *et al.* 2005). Despite this, antiviral medications have been actively promoted as a legitimate mitigation strategy by prominent virologists such as Arnold S. Monto and Frederick G. Hayden since the late 1990s (Hayden 1997, Monto 1997), and by 2005 – at the height of concern regarding the international spread of the H5N1 avian influenza virus – leading governance institutions were already widely promoting their use and stockpiling, noting that vaccines and antivirals existed as 'the two most important medical interventions for reducing illness and deaths during a pandemic' (IMF 2006, p. 12). Given that limited clinical trials had only revealed that antivirals may reduce the severity of pandemic influenza-related illness by approximately 1.5–2.5 days, and only if administered within 48 hours of the onset of symptoms (Stiver 2003, Gostin 2006), what can account for this remarkable turn of events?

Arguably, several factors help explain why drug-based interventions have been so clearly prioritised. For example, between 1997 and 2005 institutions such as the WHO, World Bank, IMF and OIE embarked on extensive campaigns to encourage governments to develop national pandemic preparedness plans (WHO 2004, Dutta 2008). In developing these plans, officials were encouraged to consider a range of mitigation strategies based on 'impartial' technical advice, and test those strategies using scenario-based exercises and/or mathematical and epidemiological modelling (Stöhr 2003). The results of such activities, which frequently described the benefits of pharmaceutical interventions over other community-based measures such as quarantine and isolation, were often published in leading scientific journals such as *Nature* and *Vaccine* by leading epidemiologists, biostatisticians, virologists and microbiologists (Longini *et al.* 2004, Ferguson *et al.* 2006), many of whom were also consulted by governments in formulating their respective pandemic plans (UK Department of Health 2011). As a result, other public health measures such as wearing face masks, hand washing and social distancing measures (e.g. school and child care centre closures and cancellation of mass gatherings) were deemed less effective. Monto has summarised this view, noting:

> none of these measures are of clear value in preventing infection, even if they could be accomplished. A principal reason little effort has been made to determine their usefulness in the interpandemic period is the usual availability of vaccine, which is of known value in prevention'. (Monto 2006, p. 55)

Said another way, drug-based measures could be quantified more easily using biostatistical techniques such as RCTs than individual or community-based interventions. When these views were further reinforced by expert authorities – both internationally respected individuals and leading global health governance institutions – combined with the political imperative for solutions generated by the international spread of the H5N1 virus and the dire warnings that another pandemic was overdue, by 2005 attention had understandably fixated on the 'proven' efficacy of vaccines and antivirals.

The political authority and problem of EBM in pandemic influenza preparedness

Frames are strategic tools that agents use to influence decision-makers and shape public policy. Importantly, frames may be deployed either intentionally or subconsciously using a variety of linguistic, cognitive, cultural or symbolic references in order to 'draw attention toward and confer legitimacy upon particular aspects of reality while marginalizing other aspects' (Lawrence 2000, p. 93). In so doing, frames (and the agents that employ them) have the ability to affect not only what people believe but also the importance that people attach to certain beliefs (Nelson and Oxley 1999). The outcome of this process is a prioritisation of issues based on peoples' beliefs and perceptions. Frames, and the agents that utilise them, can thereby wield considerable political power in the sense that they affect the way in which issues and events are perceived and interpreted, which in turn affects how decision-makers respond.

Despite the innumerable benefits generated by biomedical science and the practitioners that wield it, it is well recognised that political manipulation of science and scientific results remains a constant risk. Of course, this political manipulation can take innumerable forms – it may be inadvertent or intentional, subtle or overt, and undertaken by a variety of agents that may or may not be directly involved. Further, manipulation can occur post-event via re-interpretation, and in this sense it is not limited by temporal constraints. For instance, as Denny has observed, 'Science itself is not understood as situated or contingent knowledge; rather, it can be distorted from its ideal of objectivity by bias, which the scientist must guard against' (Denny 1999, p. 255). Haas concurs with this view, but notes that the manipulation can also be multi-directional, arguing that 'Science, in short, influences the way politics is done. Science becomes a component of politics because the scientific way of grasping reality is used to defend the interests that political actors articulate and defend' (Haas 1990, p. 11). It is in this regard that the practice whereby biomedical science is traditionally presented as apolitical is highly problematic. Moreover, even EBM, which has attempted to counter this acknowledged weakness, has similarly failed to overcome the potential of political manipulation. As Goldenberg writes:

> Because EBM is largely an effort to manage the unruly social world in which medicine is practiced via objective scientific procedure...such efforts tend to disguise political interests in the authority of so-called "scientific evidence". The configuration of policy considerations and clinical standards into questions of evidence conveniently transform normative questions into technical ones. Political issues are not resolved, however, but merely disguised in technocratic consideration and language. Thus the goals of medicine and other normative considerations lie just below the surface of these evidentiary questions, and evidence becomes an instrument of, rather than a substitute for, politics. (Goldenberg 2006, p. 2630)

Thus, despite the 'promise' of EBM being 'a more systematic and scientific practice of clinical medicine' (Tonelli 1998, p. 1234), it is argued here that how 'evidence' is presented – whether in the form of RCTs or experiential opinion – is an inherently political process. Marston and Watts summarise this best, noting 'There is nothing particular novel—or controversial—about the idea that policy should be based on evidence, but what can properly count as evidence in policy-making process *is* contentious' (Marston and Watts 2003, p. 145).[1]

As noted above, however, from the late 1990s onwards, EBM techniques, processes and methods have been systematically deployed in a range of national and international contexts to validate and inform pandemic influenza public policy. This shift came about, to a large extent, due the rationalist underpinnings that EBM encapsulates. As Denny observes, for instance, one of the reasons why the movement has spread so pervasively has been because 'The term "evidence-based medicine" has a ring of obviousness to it which makes it difficult to argue against' (Denny 1999, p. 247). In such an environment, especially when confronted with an existential threat in the form of pandemic influenza, the appeal of EBM to inform public policy is understandably strong.

The problem that emerges, however, is that by its very nature, EBM automatically biases pharmaceutical-based measures over other public health interventions such as face masks, hand washing and social distancing measures, simply because vaccines and antiviral medications can more easily be tested and evaluated by the 'gold standard' of RCTs. Moreover, as reflected by the use of terms such as 'gold standard' and 'best practice', positive values have been ascribed to the various levels of evidence generated by EBM techniques. Policies that draw on EBM-preferred levels of evidence (and particularly RCTs) are perceived as inherently better than those that do not. The intrinsic bias (and some could even argue duplicity given EBM's claim to be value-neutral) has even led some respected influenza experts to declare that 'School closure, quarantine, travel restrictions and so on are unlikely to be more effective than a garden hose in a forest fire' (Laver 2005, p. 821). This is despite the fact that a number of studies have suggested that non-pharmaceutical measures can be an effective means of limiting the spread of pandemic influenza (Kelso *et al.* 2009). As a result, organisations such as the WHO, the World Bank and UNSIC have repeatedly emphasised the need for governments to secure access to these drugs (UNSIC and World Bank 2008), even going so far as to identify them as 'desirable' (WHO 2004, p. 7), compared to the majority of non-pharmaceutical interventions that 'are based on limited evidence' (WHO 2005c, p. 18). Whether intended or not, the outcome of this practice has been to distort existing governance arrangements towards drug-based interventions. One of the more blatant examples of how this distortion has manifested transpired in late 2006.

In response to the perceived threat from the H5N1 avian influenza virus from late 2004 onwards, various governments progressively set out to secure access to antivirals and influenza vaccines by arranging advance purchase agreements (APAs) with pharmaceutical manufacturers. Indonesia, as the country worst affected by the H5N1 virus, was similarly anxious to gain access to such drugs, but by the time Indonesia's president authorised the requisite diversion of funds to arrange a national stockpile, they confronted a queue. Soon thereafter, in late 2006 an Australian pharmaceutical manufacturer developed an influenza vaccine using samples that Indonesia had supplied to the WHO without the Indonesian authorities' permission. Indonesia's inability to access these drugs, despite having provided the original genetic material, prompted the health minister to announce in December 2006 that her government would cease sharing H5N1 virus samples with the WHO in an attempt to force a fundamental restructuring of existing governance mechanisms (Sedyaningsih *et al.* 2008). Not surprisingly, Indonesia's actions immediately prompted widespread condemnation (Fidler 2010), and although an agreement was eventually reached in the form of the *2011 Pandemic Influenza*

Preparedness Framework, settling the diplomatic impasse took considerable political capital and over 4 years to resolve (Kamradt-Scott and Lee 2011, WHO 2011b).

The distortion to contemporary governance arrangements generated by the focus on vaccines and antivirals becomes particularly apparent when considering at least four additional factors as well. It is interesting to note, for instance, that other pharmaceutical measures such as statins (drugs that are usually used to lower cholesterol and prevent heart disease) have been effectively ignored as a potential influenza treatment, despite promising clinical trial results that indicate statins could be useful in reducing influenza morbidity and mortality (Fedson 2009, Vandermeer *et al.* 2012). Although the application of statin-based treatment strategies for influenza-related illness should be approached with legitimate caution, if accurate, this apparent omission is difficult to reconcile given the acknowledged limitation of existing antivirals in reducing influenza-related illness, and the accessibility and comparative low cost of statins. A second factor to note is that while much of the focus has remained on vaccines and antivirals, considerably less attention has been accorded to improving the evidence base for non-pharmaceutical measures, even though such measures are recognised as probably the most important for low- and middle-income countries (LMICs) (Oshitani *et al.* 2008, UNSIC and World Bank 2008). Instead, high-income countries have allocated and spent literally billions of dollars procuring large stockpiles of antivirals, and arranging APAs with pharmaceutical manufacturers to enable priority access to pandemic-specific vaccine supplies (GSK 2007, Third World Network 2007). Arguably, however, some of the most disturbing revelations relate to the 2009 H1N1 influenza pandemic.

Indeed, further exemplifying the weight afforded to pharmaceutical interventions within pandemic preparedness, in 2009, of the estimated US$1.48 billion needed to support 95 of the least-resourced countries, some US$1.14 billion – or 77% – was allocated to purchasing 'H1N1 vaccines and other medicines' (UNSIC and World Bank 2010, p. 30). Within days of the WHO Director-General declaring the outbreak in Mexico, attention had shifted to the capacity of pharmaceutical manufacturers to produce vaccines and the shortfall that would ensue due to global demand (Cohen and Enserink 2009). Soon thereafter, pressure began to mount on pharmaceutical companies to convert from manufacturing seasonal influenza vaccines to producing a pandemic-specific version, even though it was acknowledged that such action may cause unintended deaths due to shortages in seasonal vaccine availability (Collin *et al.* 2009). Medical professionals were, perhaps quite understandably and reasonably, at the centre of these debates, advising governments (Tay *et al.* 2010), reviewing and publishing a range of preliminary epidemiological studies that predicted the potential case fatality rates and impact of the outbreak in respected scientific journals such as *Science*, *Vaccine* and *Nature* (Fraser *et al.* 2009), and advocating that 'Programs for greater efficiency in producing effective and safe influenza vaccines have been too long delayed in development and need to be implemented quickly, to assure that this and future threats of pandemic influenza can be met' (Gallaher 2009, p. 6). Somewhat ironically though, the speed with which pharmaceutical manufacturers produced a H1N1-specific vaccine became an important factor affecting public trust and the uptake of vaccines (Steelfischer *et al.* 2010). Rather than questioning the strategy to rapidly produce vaccines, in the wake of the 2009 pandemic attention has instead shifted (at least in some sectors) to how medical experts and government officials can more effectively communicate public messages of vaccine safety, on the assumption that better evidence communicated appropriately will result in greater uptake (Brown *et al.* 2010).

In fact if it is accepted, as has been argued above, that EBM has been an important tool in shaping – and somewhat distorting – not only pandemic influenza public policy but also the world's influenza governance arrangements and institutions, the question that inevitably arises from this analysis is who benefits from this arrangement? The seemingly obvious answer to this question is the pharmaceutical companies that produce influenza vaccines and antiviral medications; yet while legitimate questions emerge about the role of some senior US government officials who possess financial links with the manufacturers of oseltamivir (Tamiflu®) (Jack 2009), this conclusion ignores the reality that historically, manufacturing influenza vaccines remains a low-profit industry (Sheridan 2005). Rather, within high-income countries the benefits of the EBM framing exercise have been (and arguably remain) much more diversified, extending to a wide variety of actors, which may also explain its apparent success.

For example, elected officials have benefited from the EBM movement as it has allowed them, when confronted with an existential threat in the form of pandemic influenza, to justify expending scarce resources in purchasing statistically validated, proven means of protecting their respective populations, thereby fulfilling the terms of the social contract between state and citizen. Likewise EBM, which offers the promise of rationalist policy-making, grants policy-makers the ability to make recommendations based on purportedly independent, scientific and impartial data, which in turn reduces their professional risk. As Wilkinson has observed, this is because rationalist policy-making extricates 'values from the policy process, prescribing an ideal type of policy making whereby the personal beliefs of policy makers and the values of society at large can be either removed or reduced to externalities' (Wilkinson 2011, p. 960). Medical professionals, which have become the proverbial guardians of the EBM movement, have similarly benefitted, for, as Denny notes:

> EBM can be understood as an attempt to re-enforce and re-regulate the medical authority of medical doctors in relation to patients, other health professions, and practitioners of complementary therapies; and to maintain a hard won status of privilege and authority in a broader social context. (Denny 1999, pp. 247–248)

In addition, the focus on vaccines and antivirals has given medical experts a greater role in contributing to national security policy (see Elbe 2011). Even in spite of the reportedly low profit margin, pharmaceutical companies have also benefitted to some degree by EBM's verification of influenza vaccines and antivirals, as it has reaffirmed the importance of drug-based treatments to society; and last, but not the least, the general public within high-income countries has benefitted from the EBM movement as it has reaffirmed the importance of a particular type of healthcare intervention – namely pharmaceuticals – as well as a measure of physical and psychological security.

Yet, whereas various actors within high-income countries benefit from this situation, a very different picture emerges within those countries that are unable to purchase the 'gold-standard' drug-based solutions. Low-income countries have been particularly disadvantaged by the EBM-driven focus on vaccines and antivirals, in large part because of the corresponding impact this emphasis has had on discouraging more research into building the evidence base for non-pharmaceutical measures. The lack of effort – and in some instances, even derision – of other interventions such as social distancing measures (e.g. cancellation of mass gatherings and school closures) and personal protection techniques (e.g. hand washing) has been particularly disturbing from a public health perspective, if for no other reason than the fact that these measures may be more appropriate for countries that lack the financial means to purchase large quantities of influenza-related pharmaceuticals. In so doing, by prioritising vaccines and antivirals, EBM has failed to meet the needs of the world's poorest and underprivileged – an outcome that is undoubtedly at odds with the humanitarian objectives often associated with medicine.

Having said this, it is again important to stress that EBM is simply a tool – it is not the cause of the world's ills, nor equally, can it be the saviour. It would be erroneous to suggest, for example, that EBM is solely responsible for empowering and validating the political authority of some actors on the one hand, while conversely disempowering and disenfranchising other groups of stakeholders on the other. Lack of access to life-saving pharmaceutical treatments was a significant problem well before the introduction of EBM, and it is likely to remain an ongoing challenge for many years to come. The key issue, however, is that through its techniques, methods and knowledge that preferences pharmaceutical-based solutions EBM has arguably served to exacerbate the divisions, making the schism between the 'haves' and the 'have nots' more stark while doing little to bridge the divide.

Conclusion

The global dissemination of the EBM movement over the past 20 years has effectively revolutionised the way in which politicians, policy-makers, and health practitioners develop and implement health-related public policy. According to Mykhalovskiy and Weir, this is principally because 'EBM has grown into one of the most important and successful initiatives to recompose contemporary biomedical reasoning and practice' (Mykhalovskiy and Weir 2004, pp. 1059–1060). Even so, and while there are undoubtedly several advantages to employing EBM-related techniques and knowledge, as this article has attempted to highlight in relation to pandemic influenza preparedness, there have also been a number of unintended, undesirable consequences. Foremost amongst these has been the preoccupation that has developed with influenza vaccines and antiviral medications as the most appropriate public health intervention to prevent, control and treat pandemic influenza. While this fixation with pharmaceutical-based measures did not originate with EBM, the techniques, processes and knowledge that EBM utilises automatically preferences drug-based solutions.

Indeed, the gradual, unrelenting emphasis on vaccines since the 1950s as the ultimate instrument in the fight against influenza, combined with the securitisation of the disease in the late twentieth century and the deployment of EBM as a legitimating tool, has served to overly politicise, and eventually, ultimately, destabilise the post-WWII influenza governance arrangements. Moreover, the intense focus on specific pharmaceutical measures has structured the allocation (and subsequent expenditure) of billions of dollars in public funding on interventions that debatably benefit a comparatively small proportion of humankind located primarily in high-income countries. In the event that another pandemic of similar lethality to the 1918 Spanish Influenza was to occur, and the world is to be better prepared to defend itself, a rebalancing of the current governance and funding arrangements is conceivably required. What this rebalancing would entail in practice is open to debate, but at the very minimum it would involve some discussion of, and ideally prompt further research into, the use of alternative, non-pharmaceutical measures to inform pandemic influenza public policy. Until such investigations are undertaken and the effectiveness of non-pharmaceutical measures is more comprehensively assessed, it is likely that very little will change, and those who have consistently been at the greatest risk of high morbidity and mortality from pandemic influenza – namely, the world's poorest – will suffer the most.

Acknowledgements

This research has been made possible through funding from the European Research Council under the European Community's Seventh Framework Programme – Ideas Grant 230489 GHG. Thanks are also extended to the two anonymous reviewers, and to Colin McInnes and Kelley Lee for their helpful comments. All views expressed remain those of the author.

Note

1. Italics in original.

References

Boswell, C., 2009. *The political uses of expert knowledge: immigration policy and social research.* Cambridge: Cambridge University Press.

Brown, K.F., Kroll, J.S., Hudson, M.J., Ramsay, M., Green, J., Vincent, C.A., Fraser, G., and Sevdalis, N., 2010. Omission bias and vaccine rejection by parents of healthy children: implications for the influenza A/H1N1 vaccination programme. *Vaccine*, 28 (25), 4181–4185.

Cohen, J. and Enserink, M., 2009. As swine flu circles globe, scientists grapple with basic questions. *Science*, 324 (5927), 572–573.

Collin, N., Radiguès, X., and WHO H1N1 Vaccine Task Force, 2009. Vaccine production capacity for seasonal and pandemic (H1N1) 2009 influenza. *Vaccine*, 27 (38), 5184–5186.

Davidoff, F., Haynes, B., Sackett, D., and Smith, R., 1995. Evidence based medicine. *British Medical Journal*, 310 (6987), 1085–1086.

Denny, K., 1999. Evidence-based medicine and medical authority. *Journal of Medical Humanities*, 20 (4), 247–263.

Department of Health (UK), 2011. *Scientific pandemic influenza advisory committee (SPI)* [online]. Available from: http://www.dh.gov.uk/ab/SPI/DH_095670 [Accessed 16 September 2011].

Dobbie, A.E., Schneider, D.F., Anderson, A.D., and Littlefield, J., 2000. What evidence supports teaching evidence-based medicine? *Academic Medicine*, 75 (12), 1184–1185.

Dutta, A., 2008. *The effectiveness of policies to control a human influenza pandemic: a literature review Policy research working paper 4524.* Washington, DC: World Bank.

Elbe, S., 2011. Pandemics on the radar screen: health security, infectious disease and the medicalisation of insecurity. *Political Studies*, 59 (4), 848–866.

Fedson, D., 2009. Meeting the challenge of influenza pandemic preparedness in developing countries. *Emerging Infectious Diseases*, 15 (3), 365–371.

Ferguson, N.M., Cummings, D.A., Fraser, C., Cajka, J.C., Cooley, P.C., and Burke, D.S., 2006. Strategies for mitigating an influenza pandemic. *Nature*, 442 (7101), 448–452.

Fidler, D., 2010. Negotiating equitable access to influenza vaccines: global health diplomacy and the controversies surrounding avian influenza H5N1 and pandemic influenza H1N1. *Public Library of Science Medicine*, 7 (5), 1–4.

Francis, T., 1947. A consideration of vaccination against influenza. *The Milbank Memorial Fund Quarterly*, 25 (1), 5–10.

Fraser, C., Donnelly, C.A., Cauchemez, S., Hanage, W.P., Van Kerkhove, M.D., Hollingsworth, D.T., Griffin, J., Baggaley, R.F., Jenkins, H.E., Lyons, E.J., Jombart, T., Hinsley, W.R., Grassly, N.C., Balloux, F., Ghani, A.C., Ferguson, N.M., Rambaut, A., Pybus, O.G., Lopez-Gatell, H., Alpuche-Aranda, C.M., Bojorquez Chapela, L., Palacios Zavala, E., Espejo Guevara, D.M., Checchi, F., Garcia, E., Hugonnet, S., Roth, C., and Rapid Pandemic Assessment Collaboration, WHO, 2009. Pandemic potential of a strain of influenza A (H1N1): early findings. *Science*, 324 (5934), 1557–1561.

Gallaher, W., 2009. *Towards a sane and rational approach to management of Influenza H1N1 2009* [online]. Available from: http://www.virologyj.com/content/6/1/51 [Accessed 14 December 2011].

Goldenberg, M., 2006. On evidence and evidence-based medicine: lessons from the philosophy of science. *Social Science and Medicine*, 62 (11), 2621–2632.

Gostin, L.O., 2006. Medical countermeasures for pandemic influenza: ethics and the law. *Journal of the American Medical Association*, 295 (5), 554–556.

GSK, 2007. *New studies indicate GSK's pre-pandemic influenza vaccine can protect against different strains of H5N1* [online]. Available from: http://www.gsk.com/media/pressreleases/2007/2007_03_05_GSK989.htm [Accessed 16 September 2011].

Haas, E.B., 1990. *When knowledge is power: three models of change in international organizations*. London: University of California Press.

Hayden, F.G., 1997. Antivirals for pandemic influenza. *Journal of Infectious Diseases*, 176 (Suppl. 1), S56–S61.

Hota, S. and McGeer, A., 2007. Antivirals and the control of influenza outbreaks. *Clinical Infectious Diseases*, 45 (10), 1362–1368.

IMF, 2006. *The global economic and financial impact of an avian flu pandemic and the role of the IMF* [online]. Washington, DC: International Monetary Fund. Available from: http://www.imf.org/external/pubs/ft/afp/2006/eng/022806.pdf [Accessed 24 February 2011].

Jack, A., 2009. Flu's unexpected bonus. *British Medical Journal*, 339, b3811.

Jensen, K. and Hogan, R., 1958. Laboratory diagnosis of Asian influenza. *Public Health Reports (1896–1970)*, 73 (2), 140–144.

Kamradt-Scott, A., 2012. Changing perceptions of pandemic influenza and public health responses. *American Journal of Public Health Policy*, 102 (1), 90–98.

Kamradt-Scott, A., forthcoming. The politics of medicine and the global governance of pandemic influenza. *International Journal of Health Services*.

Kamradt-Scott, A. and Lee, K., 2011. The 2011 pandemic influenza preparedness framework: global health secured or a missed opportunity? *Political Studies*, 59 (4), 831–847.

Kelso, J., Milne, G., and Kelly, H., 2009. *Simulation suggests that rapid activation of social distancing can arrest epidemic development due to a novel strain of influenza* [online]. Available from: http://www.biomedcentral.com/1471-2458/9/117 [Accessed 25 February 2011].

Kitler, M., Gavinio, P., and Lavanchy, D., 2002. Influenza and the work of the World Health Organization. *Vaccine*, 20 (Suppl. 2), S5–S14.

Kristiansen, I.S. and Mooney, G., 2004. Evidence-based medicine: method, collaboration, movement or crusade? *In*: I.S. Kristiansen and G. Mooney, eds. *Evidence-based medicine: in its place*. Abingdon: Routledge, 1–19 (Chapter 1).

Lawrence, R.G., 2000. Game-framing the issues: tracking the strategy frame in public policy news. *Political Communication*, 17, 93–114.

Laver, G., 2005. Influenza drug could abort a pandemic. *Nature*, 434 (7035), 821.

Lederberg, J., 1996. Infectious disease—a threat to global health and security. *Journal of the American Medical Association*, 276 (5), 417–419.

Longini, I.M., Halloran, M.E., Nizam, A., and Yang, Y., 2004. Containing pandemic influenza with antiviral agents. *American Journal of Epidemiology*, 159 (7), 623–633.

MacPhail, T., 2009. The politics of bird flu: the battle over virus samples and China's role in global public health. *Journal of Language and Politics*, 8 (3), 456–475.

Marston, G. and Watts, R., 2003. Tampering with the evidence: a critical appraisal of evidence-based policy-making. *The Drawing Board: An Australian Review of Public Affairs*, 3 (3), 143–163.

Monto, A.S., 1997. Prospects for pandemic influenza control with currently available vaccines and antivirals. *Journal of Infectious Diseases*, 176 (Suppl. 1), S32–S37.

Monto, A.S., 2006. Vaccines and antiviral drugs in pandemic preparedness. *Emerging Infectious Diseases*, 12 (1), 55–60.

Mykhalovskiy, E. and Weir, L., 2004. The problem of evidence-based medicine: directions for social science. *Social Science and Medicine*, 59 (5), 1059–1069.

Nelson, T.E. and Oxley, Z.M., 1999. Issue framing effects on belief importance and opinion. *Journal of Politics*, 61 (4), 1040–1067.

Nichol, K., Lind, A., Margolis, K., Murdoch, M., McFadden, R., Hauge, R., Magnan, S., and Drake, M., 1995. The effectiveness of vaccination against influenza in healthy, working adults. *New England Journal of Medicine*, 333 (14), 889–893.

Oshitani, H., Kamigaki, T., and Suzuki, A., 2008. Major issues and challenges of influenza pandemic preparedness in developing countries. *Emerging Infectious Diseases*, 14 (6), 875–880.

Payne, A., 1953. The influenza programme of WHO. *Bulletin of the World Health Organization*, 8 (5–6), 755–792.

Pereira, M.S., 1979. Global surveillance of influenza. *British Medical Bulletin*, 35 (1), 9–14.

Pope, C., 2003. Resisting evidence: the study of evidence-based medicine as a contemporary social movement. *Health*, 7 (3), 267–282.

Ruben, F., 1987. Prevention and control of influenza: role of vaccine. *American Journal of Medicine*, 82 (6) (Suppl. 1), 31–34.

Sackett, D. and Rosenberg, W., 1995. The need for evidence-based medicine. *Journal of the Royal Society for Medicine*, 88, 620–624.

Sedyaningsih, E.R., Isfandari, S., Soendoro, T., and Supari, S.F., 2008. Towards mutual trust, transparency and equity in virus sharing mechanism: the avian influenza case of Indonesia. *Annals Academy of Medicine*, 37 (6), 482–488.

Sheridan, C., 2005. The business of making vaccines. *Nature Biotechnology*, 23 (11), 1359–1366.

Shuchman, M., 2007. Improving global health—Margaret Chan at the WHO. *New England Journal of Medicine*, 356 (7), 653–656.

Smith, A., 1996. Mad cows and ecstasy: chance and choice in an evidence-based society. *Journal of the Royal Statistical Society: Series A*, 159 (3), 367–383.

Snacken, R., Kendal, A., Haaheim, L., and Wood, J., 1999. The next influenza pandemic: lessons from Hong Kong, 1997. *Emerging Infectious Diseases*, 5 (2), 195–203.

Steelfischer, G.K., Blendon, R.J., Bekheit, M.M., and Lubell, K., 2010. The public's response to the 2009 H1N1 influenza pandemic. *New England Journal of Medicine*, 362 (22), 65.

Stiver, G., 2003. The treatment of influenza with antiviral drugs. *Canadian Medical Association Journal*, 168 (1), 49–56.

Stöhr, K., 2003. The global agenda on influenza surveillance and control. *Vaccine*, 21 (16), 1744–1748.

Tay, J., Ng, Y.F., Cutter, J., and James, L., 2010. Influenza A (H1N1–2009) pandemic in Singapore—public health control measures implemented and lessons learnt. *Annals Academy of Medicine Singapore*, 39 (4), 313–324.

Third World Network, 2007. *Winners and losers in the sharing of avian flu viruses* [online]. Available from: http://www.twnside.org.sg/title2/intellectual_property/info.service/twn.ipr. info.050705.htm [Accessed 16 September 2011].

Tonelli, M., 1998. The philosophical limits of evidence-based medicine. *Academic Medicine*, 73 (12), 1234–1240.

UNSIC and World Bank, 2008. *Responses to avian influenza and state of pandemic readiness. Third global progress report*, December 2007. New York: United Nations System Influenza Coordination.

UNSIC and World Bank. 2010. *Animal and pandemic influenza: a framework for sustaining momentum. Fifth global progress report*, July 2010. New York: United Nations System Influenza Coordination.

Vandermeer, M., Thomas, A., Kamimoto, K., Reingold, A., Gershman, K., Meek, J., Farley, M., Ryan, P., Lynfield, R., Baumbach, J., Schaffner, W., Bennett, N., and Zansky, S., 2012. Association between use of statins and mortality among patients hospitalized with laboratory-confirmed influenza virus infections: a multistate study. *Journal of Infectious Diseases*, 205 (1), 13–19.

Ward, P., Small, I., Smith, J., Suter, P., and Dutkowski, R., 2005. Osteltamivir (Tamiflu®) and its potential for use in the event of an influenza pandemic. *Journal of Antimicrobial Chemotherapy*, 55 (Suppl. 1), i5–i121.

Webster, R., 1994. While awaiting the next pandemic of influenza. *British Medical Journal*, 309 (6063), 1179.

Webster, R. and Kawaoka, Y., 1994. Influenza—an emerging and re-emerging disease. *Virology*, 5 (2), 103–111.

Wilkinson, K., 2011. Organised chaos: an interpretive approach to evidence-based policy making in Defra. *Political Studies*, 59 (4), 959–977.

WHO, 1988. Consultation with directors of WHO collaborating centres on influenza: memorandum from a WHO meeting. *Bulletin of the World Health Organization*, 66 (4), 457–458.

WHO, 1994. Emerging infectious diseases: memorandum from a WHO meeting. *Bulletin of the World Health Organization*, 72 (6), 845–850.

WHO, 1999. *Influenza pandemic preparedness plan: the role of WHO and guidelines for national and regional planning, Geneva, Switzerland, April 1999*. Geneva: World Health Organization.

WHO, 2004. *WHO influenza pandemic preparedness checklist* [online]. Geneva: World Health Organization. Available from: http://www.wpro.who.int/internet/resources.ashx/CSR/Publications/WHO + Influenza + Pandemic + Preparedness + Checklist.pdf [Accessed 24 February 2011].

WHO, 2005a. *Avian influenza: assessing the pandemic threat* [online]. Geneva: World Health Organization. Available from: http://www.who.int/csr/disease/influenza/H5N1–9reduit.pdf [Accessed 22 February 2011].

WHO, 2005b. *WHO global influenza preparedness plan: the role of WHO and recommendations for national measures before and during pandemics* [online]. Geneva: World Health Organization. Available from: http://whqlibdoc.who.int/hq/2005/WHO_CDS_CSR_GIP_2005.5.pdf [Accessed 1 December 2011].

WHO, 2005c. *WHO checklist for influenza pandemic preparedness planning* [online]. Geneva: World Health Organization. Available from: http://www.who.int/csr/resources/publications/influenza/FluCheck6web.pdf [Accessed 25 February 2011].

WHO. 2009. *Pandemic influenza preparedness and response: a WHO guidance document* [online]. Geneva: World Health Organization. Available from: http://www.who.int/influenza/resources/documents/pandemic_guidance_04_2009/en/index.html [Accessed 2 May 2012].

WHO, 2011a. *WHO global influenza surveillance network* [online]. Available from: http://www.who.int/csr/disease/influenza/surveillance/en/index.html [Accessed 18 February 2011].

WHO, 2011b. *Pandemic influenza preparedness framework for the sharing of influenza viruses and access to vaccines and other benefits* [online]. Available from: www.who.int/csr/disease/influenza/pip_framework_16_april_2011.pdf [Accessed 11 September 2011].

Access to medicines, market failure and market intervention: A tale of two regimes

Owain D. Williams

Department of International Politics, Centre for Health and International Relations, Aberystwyth University, Aberystwyth, UK

This study explores how an 'Intellectual Property Rights (IPR)/trade regime' has generated a particular set of problems regarding access to medicines despite patents on drugs being presented as economically necessary for reward and future drug innovation. These problems have also inspired and informed activities by so-called new actors in global health. This study argues that a parallel 'pro-access regime' has developed in order to correct some of the most high-profile issues associated with a dysfunctional global pharmaceutical market, especially problems regarding price and innovation that have been exacerbated by stringent global patent rights on new drugs. Therefore, the IPR/trade regime's basic role in global-health governance diverges from how it has been framed and understood, not least of all by its constituent agents and donors. The pro-access regime encompasses new actors in health such as Global Health Partnerships (e.g., GAVI Alliance and the Global Fund to Fight AIDS, Tuberculosis and Malaria), major philanthropic foundations (e.g., the Gates and Clinton Foundations) and new access initiatives (e.g., UNITAID). The study problematises these actors' governance roles with respect to the overarching authority of the IPR/trade regime and makes a case that the two regimes should be understood as being closely connected with respect to the governance of access to medicines and the global political economy of pharmaceuticals.

Introduction

Access to medicines has emerged in recent decades as a totemic problem in global health. Approximately one-third (or roughly 2 billion) of the world's population lacks access to drugs (UN Millennium Project 2005). However, they are afflicted by, or even die from, diseases that are either preventable or curable, or they suffer each day from often debilitating and painful symptoms of disease that can be managed and ameliorated by existing treatments. In other cases, no drugs have yet been created for certain diseases, and people suffer or die. This is often because they are too poor to provide an adequate economic incentive for biomedical research and development (R&D) of new medicines for their particular disease burden. Access to medicines is therefore clearly one of the most pressing and morally compelling problems we face as humanity.

While HIV/AIDS has served to crystallise many of the issues associated with access to medicines and has spurred the creation of numerous initiatives to increase the supply of antiretroviral treatments (ARTs), it is still the case that only 54% of those who need them have access to those treatments (UNAIDS 2012). For other diseases (especially tropical and waterborne diseases), the problem of access is even more acute (Ravvin 2008). Often, no drugs or formulations exist to treat these diseases even though the pathologies of some of these diseases have been known for decades. There has been a failure, and some would say a market failure (Kremer 2002, Rosiello and Smith 2004), to incentivise the necessary R&D to generate appropriate drugs. In global terms, this failure in the system of pharmaceutical innovation has been labelled the 90/10 gap, in which 90% of pharmaceutical and biomedical R&D is targeted at just 10% of the global burden of disease (Troullier *et al.* 2002).

This study examines how we have sought to 'govern our way out' of the problem of access to medicines and does so by providing an overview of the activities of the new health initiatives and partnerships that are addressing this issue. The most prominent of these actors are Global Health Partnerships (GHPs), new and old philanthropic foundations (Rushton and Williams 2011), and a raft of more specialised initiatives targeted at medical product R&D, often involving hybrid public/private forms of research and project collaboration. These actors are rarely analysed as being primarily associated with access to medicines, nor are they viewed as having, in essence, a common function of intervening in global pharmaceutical markets. Nonetheless, this study forwards the case that at a very basic level, widening access to medicines represents a fundamental and central pillar of their activities, and that these actors seek to correct some of the problems regarding access that are associated with a dysfunctional global pharmaceutical market. They do so either by facilitating lower drug prices for select diseases, by financing their purchase at the level of donor–recipient countries, by blocking procurement of certain treatments or by stimulating R&D for neglected diseases and other areas. Market intervention is therefore viewed as being both a core programmatic and policy objective of what this study labels a 'pro-access' regime, and it supplies the basis for understanding how this regime should be considered within the broader landscape of contemporary governance and the political economy of pharmaceutical innovation, production and price. As indicated earlier, the actors that constitute the pro-access regime include new GHPs such as the Global Fund to Fight AIDS, Tuberculosis and Malaria (the Global Fund) and the Global Alliance for Vaccines and Immunization (GAVI); bilateral platforms and programmes for access such as the US President's Emergency Plan for AIDS Relief (PEPFAR); new specialised initiatives for medical R&D such as the Drugs for Neglected Diseases Initiative (DNDi); as well as philanthropic actors in health like the Clinton and Gates foundations.

The role of new actors and initiatives in global health are viewed as having many positive elements with respect to widening access to medicines, but this role is also deeply problematic and poorly understood with respect to the negative outcomes that the global political economy of pharmaceuticals continues to produce. Indeed, despite bringing vast resources to bear on the problem of access (Ravishankar *et al.* 2009), the new actors in global health are neither the only nor the most important actors engaged in access to medicines. While we should view the new initiatives, partnerships and foundations as constituting a new modality of health governance,

and as having brought new sets of policies and practices to secure access to medicines (Rushton and Williams 2011), they are best understood as being only *one of two* major regimes governing and determining outcomes in the area. In fact, these new actors operate in the context of a cluster of agreements, rules, institutions and actors associated with international trade and Intellectual Property Rights (IPR) (a regime especially associated with the World Trade Organization (WTO) and a series of bilateral, regional and new plurilateral trade-related initiatives; the developed countries and firms that promote them; and the establishment of stringent and globalised patent rights for medicines and other technologies). The pro-access regime is therefore considered as being reactive and only partially corrective to some of the negative outcomes this IPR/trade regime has generated in regard to drug prices and innovation.

The central thesis of this study is, therefore, that these two regimes are on some levels fundamentally connected with each other, not least of all in their response to basic (economic) problems associated with markets as they relate to drug prices and innovation. Although the new actors and initiatives associated with the pro-access regime ostensibly have a different function or starting point with regard to the problems of access, providing rhetorical and practical support toward increasing drug availability, they have failed to challenge the underlying economic rationale for strict and global drug patents. Moreover, in some ways their very presence has given the IPR/trade regime an opportunity to reconsolidate, and helped offer it new legitimacy after a period of sustained attacks with regard to its negative impact on drug access

This study argues that while the framing of drug patenting has been counter-framed by rights-based development and public-health discourses (Helfer 2004), and more recently by critical economic arguments that have confronted the core economic assumptions that justify the IPR/trade regime (Hollis 2004), the basic economic frame and ideas that have supported the globalisation of patent rights for pharmaceuticals has proven both powerful and durable. While there exists no single or coherent school or version of economics associated with such justifications, the proponents of strong IPRs have been able to appeal to common sense assumptions about the necessity of protecting pharmaceutical inventive activity in order to capture and maintain the social benefits of private innovation. The IPR/trade regime has therefore been presented as a global regulatory means to prevent the 'failure' in innovation that would otherwise occur without the presence of patents.

At the same time, the pro-access regime and its donors and supporters have generally failed to frame its role as being one of market intervention. Also, they have not problematised the contradictions of their work in the context of a monolithic IPR/trade regime. While these actors routinely frame their activities in terms of rights, public goods, development or humanitarian duty, these frames are not deployed in a manner that constitutes a concerted challenge the economic justification of drug patents, nor the wider global political economy of pharmaceutical production and innovation. This is perhaps unsurprising as many of the principal donors, collaborative partners and supporters of the pro-access regime are often archsupporters and promoters of stronger and globalised IPRs, and this crosscutting power over two regimes has effectively served to silence many of the criticisms of the IPR/trade regime from institutions that deal with the sharp end of many of the problems it produces. In this sense, many of the new partnerships, such

as GAVI Alliance and the Global Fund, do not really often exercise governance agency in a rule changing or transformational sense but are themselves governed by other agents and donors who seek either to maintain the status quo or even higher levels of IPR protection.

The first part of this study briefly explains some of the fundamental economic problems that characterise pharmaceutical production, innovation and drug markets. While all IPR regimes (and specifically here patents) seek to respond to a basic economic problem associated with knowledge production under market conditions, their interaction with pharmaceutical markets creates further sets of problems for access to medicines. Despite the disastrous impact on peoples' access to drugs, proponents of the IPR/trade regime have consistently used what are often very simple economic arguments to frame strong global patents on drugs as a positive force for drug development, and ultimately for the availability of new and improved medicines in developing countries.

The second part of this study then details many of the new actors associated with the pro-access regime and explores how they have rhetorically framed and understood their function in global health. While their role in intervening in a dysfunctional global pharmaceutical market is rarely present in their policy documentation, or indeed in their major donors' rationales for support, an assessment of some of their core activities with respect to drug price and innovation seeks to reveal that intervention is too common and fundamental an activity to be discounted. Conclusions are offered as to the nature and ramifications of the interaction of these two ostensibly discrete regimes.

The IPR/trade regime and its framing

The IPR/trade regime responds to a fundamental economic problem associated with the production of knowledge (and knowledge-based goods such as drugs) that arises from its non-rivalrous nature and the ease with which it can be copied and replicated after its invention (Stiglitz 1999, 2007). This generates a social need to reward invention in order to ensure there are economic and social incentives for the generation of future knowledge. The prevention of duplication (and free-riding) and the need to provide incentives for innovation provide the basic starting points in the argument stating that IPRs are appropriate and necessary legal frameworks to achieve these objectives (Drahos 2003; Stiglitz 2007, 2008).

This framing of IPR systems as a solution to a fundamental economic problem has characterised their social role and evolution in various early industrialising countries, and the presence of these systems are often held to be a key to the technological and economic progress enjoyed by the Global North (Braga 1989). In creating such systems, governments were essentially attempting to capture a balance between the private right of the inventor to receive rewards and the wider public good. Yet pharmaceutical patents are perhaps *the* classic example of a technology that many countries chose to exclude from their patent laws because of the competition between the social value placed on human health and the primacy of public rights in this particular balance of rights (Lanjouw 1998). Indeed, even many developed countries were notably late in adopting patent laws for drugs exactly because of these rationales (Drahos and Braithwaite 2002).

The 1994 World Trade Organization's Agreement in Trade-Related Aspects of Intellectual Property Rights (TRIPS) served to globally 'harmonise' IPR laws, including patents, making rights available in all WTO member countries, and subject to that organisation's powerful dispute-settlement body. For patents, a term of 20 years of protection was awarded (surpassing the duration then available even in the legal systems of many developed countries), and the agreement made patents available for 'all fields of technology' (WTO 1994) and for all processes for production of such technologies. Crucially, the agreement specifically included medicines and biotechnological products and processes (and indeed plant varieties) and severely limited the so-called 'flexibilities' that member countries could exercise to obviate patent rights in either special or sovereignly determined circumstances. These limitations were subject to a challenge in the WTO's 2001 Doha Declaration (WTO 2001, Abbott 2002).

TRIPS provided a global scope to patent rights for drugs. Scholars have traced how successive framings of the economic rationale for global IPRs (Odell and Sell 2006) as well as horizontal institutional and issue linkages (Helfer 2004, Muzaka 2010) were made to justify the new global regime. These included the linkage of IPRs to 'free' international trade and increased foreign investment in the South; the institutional shift of international IPRs from the World Intellectual Property Organiztion (WIPO) (a 'weak' regime) to the WTO (a 'strong' regime with disciplinary powers based on trade sanctions); the framing of IPRs and patents via a narrative of 'universal' private rights (Kinsella 2001, Sell and Prakash 2004); the linkage of patents to increased rates of global medical innovation (Mansfield 1986, Grabowski 2002); and the linkage of generic drugs with global piracy and counterfeiting. These framings contributed to the formation of a regime that substantially eroded the treatment of medicines as public goods. The frame of reference was shifted to a discourse of private goods whose allocation and production are subject to the global-market mechanism, with the purported benefits of that mechanism, namely, higher rates of innovation and lower prices via competition lurking in the background as supporting economic assumptions (Drahos and Braithwaite 2002).

These initial economic framings of the TRIPS agreement have recently developed new life and have been transposed to yet other ('TRIPS-plus') instruments and policy initiatives, all directed at raising the levels of protection and private rights that are available for medicines and other technologies (Drahos 2003, Sell 2011). Indeed, these framings are readily detectable in debates regarding so-called TRIPS-plus regional and bilateral trade agreements, as in initiatives such as the Anti-Counterfeiting Trade Agreement and 2009 EU customs seizures of generic drugs in transit.

Another success of the economic framing of TRIPS lay in the deceptively simple extension of economic justifications of national systems of IPRs to a global level, with an often implicit claim that they are equally necessary across global markets. In turn, rather than being presented as having negative consequences, the regime was held to herald long-term benefits in the form of a genuine basis for innovation in 'yet to' develop countries (see Braga *et al.* 2000). As I argue below, such assumptions are highly problematic for access to medicines, not least of all because the *legal treatment* of these markets as undifferentiated belies the fact that global pharmaceutical markets are in fact massively differentiated both across and within national markets

(Kremer 2002, Flynn *et al.* 2009) and also because many of the predicted benefits in terms of technology transfer and new medicines are not emerging.

The knock-on effects of the IPR/trade regime for access to medicines

TRIPS and the associated national and international instruments that make up the IPR/trade regime have interacted with and exacerbated certain problems that were already apparent with regard to the oligopolistic structure of the global pharmaceutical sector, as well as the huge inequalities in incomes both within and between pharmaceutical markets. More recently, especially in the post-Doha era (after 2001), these 'knock-on' problems have led to counter-framings of the relationship of patents with drug innovation and price, which have largely drawn on economic arguments emerging from heterodox or 'critical' economics and innovation studies (Hollis 2004, Hubbard and Love 2004, Ravvin 2008, Selgelid 2008, Pogge 2009, Hollis and Pogge 2010).

The first problem for access to medicines is the most obvious, and it relates to the prices of patented drugs. A patent confers, after all, a monopoly and the ability to set an artificially inflated price for a fixed period of time. Such prices are routinely set at rates that the poor cannot afford to pay out of pocket, and governments of developing country cannot subsidise consumption. Patented drugs are in some cases up to 400% more expensive than generic counterparts (Baker 2004). The exclusion of generic competition, which would bring down prices close to the marginal cost of production, is one of the principal functions of the patent system as it relates medicines. TRIPS and other associated agreements have either more narrowly circumscribed the opportunities for compulsory licensing by confining the flexibility largely to ARTs, or have introduced new tiers of legal complexity, closing off avenues by which generics could be introduced to markets (Johnston and Wasunna 2007), as is the case when limitations are placed on access to clinical trial data in some TRIPS-plus bilateral trade agreements (Sell 2011). These obstacles to generic entry obviously create particular problems for people who cannot afford to pay but who are nonetheless affected by an illness that an on-patent drug can prevent, cure or alleviate the symptoms of. It is certainly the case that generic entry permits competition that lowers prices, as has been the case with ARTs (Waning *et al.* 2009), but this avenue has been circumscribed.

The effects of globalising patent rights are particularly acute when we appreciate that the global pharmaceutical market is highly differentiated in terms of governments' and individuals' ability to pay high prices. Scholars have also identified that many developing countries are also highly differentiated *within* national markets (as are many developed country markets), not least of all by high levels of income inequality (Flynn *et al.* 2009). These market structures interact with patents to keep prices high. Flynn *et al.* (2009) found that in South Africa, high levels of income inequality mean that firms can target upper deciles of income earners and charge prices close to or exceeding the prices charged the markets of the developed countries without threatening (deadweight) losses from those consumers priced out of the market. In short, because of huge disparities in income, there is often no incentive to lower the prices of patented products and increase the volume of sales (Danzon and Towse 2003).

The second major knock-on problem in the interaction of IPRs with pharmaceutical markets relates to innovation. While the patent system supplies an incentive to invent in the presence of effective demand, in its absence there is no such motivation. Many scholars have noted that the world's poor often simply do not provide sufficient demand for drug firms to include them in their R&D and production strategies (Trouiller *et al.* 2002, Hollis 2004). This has been variously described as market failure (Kremer 2002) in the context of critical economic discourses about access to medicines, or as, perhaps more accurately, the problem of missing or non-markets (Rosiello and Smith 2004). Eighty per cent of the global market for drug sales lies in North America and Europe (Rosiello and Smith 2004), and this creates a clear incentive for firms to develop and target drugs for those populations and the particular diseases affecting them. Generally, this situation had led to a preponderance of drugs being developed for so-called lifestyle diseases or non-communicable diseases – such as cancers, cardiovascular diseases, diabetes and stress-related disorders.

Two clear issues arise from these knock-on problems. The first is the moral and human health hazards of leaving the development of medicines to the market mechanism alone when it is clearly not sufficient or effective in so many cases. The second issue is the framing of the global patent system as the answer to all innovation needs. It is not, and cannot be, as long as poor people and their governments fail to provide incentives to invent via their purchasing power.

Even so, the patent system can also create knock-on problems for innovation even when demand is present. Two examples of this negative influence are worth citing. It has been widely noted that the patent system provides a legal structure or criteria by which incremental innovation of medical technologies is encouraged, rather than the development of meaningful new drugs and treatments (Correa 2011). In short, companies have strategies that seek to extend patent life (and the profits gained from a product) by marginal tinkering with a drug's chemical composition or method of delivery. Likewise, others achieve similar gains by incrementally improving on existing products to gain a patent for so-called 'evergreening' and 'me-too' inventions, or by engendering legal complexity and uncertainty through the multiple and dense patenting of drugs – termed patent thickets (Barton and Emanuel 2005, Faunce and Lexchin 2007, Stiglitz 2007).

The rise of the pro-access regime and new approaches to access to medicines

As the issue of access to medicines became prominent in the wake of the 1994 TRIPS Agreement, the range of governance initiatives and new actors involved in tackling the access to medicines problem increased exponentially. As a result, a perception emerged that the authority of the IPR/trade regime with respect to access to medicines had been effectively politically neutered, and that the access issue had been substantially reframed in terms of development and global public goods (Sell 2002, Odell and Sell 2006) and/or in terms of human rights to health (Helfer 2004). Moreover, it has also become clear that many of the issues that pertain to wider drug availability are not solely associated with patented drugs, but with the price and supply of the vast majority of essential medicines which are off-patent, but this should not detract from the adverse impact of patent rights on generic entry or price.

But as TRIPS and medical patents were being challenged (and indeed as that challenge appeared to recede), new initiatives emerged in an effort to 'govern our way out' of the fallout of market failures with respect to drug innovation and price. Many of the new hybrid public–private GHPs, specialised R&D initiatives and key philanthropic foundations are essentially responding to these problems, albeit in different ways. These actors intervene in the global pharmaceutical market either with respect to drug prices (through subsidisation, negotiation or other forms of financing), or in terms of innovation and R&D, and sometimes with combinations of these two basic strategies. In doing so, they have created an elaborate and multifaceted global pro-access regime for access to medicines.

Before tracing the basic functional characteristics of the pro-access regime's responses to the economic problems of access to medicines, it is worth noting that their activities have rarely been explicitly framed in terms of supplying policy responses to market failure. Nonetheless, this basic market-intervention function with regard to access to medicines is very rarely far from the surface of framings of these new actors' governance roles. Nor are they far from the centre of at least 10 years of rapid institutional development and unprecedented financing in global health (Ravishankar *et al.* 2009). Rather than economics, it is international development that has most commonly represented the framing of their activities in increasing access to medicines.[1] The rapid emergence of the pro-access regime in the early twenty-first century was part of a wider development policy zeitgeist and was closely associated with the Millennium Development Goals (MDG). The G8 (and World Bank) played an instrumental role in the development of the new global-health governance regime, most notably via a series of high-profile summit commitments to health and development programmes, which gave birth to initiatives such as the Global Fund and GAVI. The major donor involvement in these organisations clearly set out a template for what these agencies would do in global health, and their governance role therein was largely predetermined. These new institutions were presented as providing the basis for an essential 'step-up' toward (economic) development and poverty alleviation (see Woodling *et al.*, this volume) through select disease interventions and not as focal points for change in the underlying political economy of pharmaceutical production and innovation.

However, the new actors and initiatives have not only framed their activities in terms of MDG-directed development, but they have also portrayed themselves as representing a new modality of health and aid (Rushton and Williams 2011). While being part of the wider state-funded and multilateral drive to development, both GHPs and foundations have sought to involve and draw upon the expertise, management skills, reporting and accounting practices as well as the best practices of a range of stakeholders, and most prominently the private sector (Rushton and Williams 2011). In particular, close collaboration with pharmaceutical firms is viewed as central to the success of the model. Industry representatives have been incorporated into both foundations and GHPs, and a revolving door of personnel has emerged between many of the institutions and drug companies. Furthermore, their programmes have often needed to produce results in short order, not least of all to satisfy donors and lend themselves output legitimacy. These pressures have further entrenched the pivotal status of widening the medicines' coverage in the disease areas they respond to, also reflecting the technical and biomedical bias embedded in the MDG health blueprint, and a basic belief in the power of the pharmaceutical sector to supply magic-bullet fixes to health problems, given the right amount of stimulus and incentive (Black *et al.* 2009). Thus 'success' for the pro-access regime has been framed in terms of the necessary involvement of pharmaceutical firms. Even though reliance on their products is not a central component of their programmes, they are still viewed as crucial to innovation and as the necessary source of original products for generic-based programmes. In key disease areas, such as HIV/AIDS and malaria, there has been a gradual shift to a greater reliance on the generic sector. However, more widely there is a tangible focus on innovator firms as either key partners in publicly funded R&D programmes or as the sole sources of drug supply when generic medications are not yet present (Youde 2011).

Finally, part of the reason for the twenty-first century surge in new institutions and health financing has clearly been ideational, and indeed resulted partly from arguments and counter-frames used to challenge the IPR-trade regime, especially in the period between the commencement of the TRIPS agreement and 2001 (the year that saw the creation of both the Doha Declaration and the Millennium Declaration) (Sell 2002). The civil society, patient groups and developing states involved in the counter-framing of the IPR/trade regime as negatively impacting either human rights or the public goods qualities of drugs (the latter frame highlighting that there are compelling moral, epidemiological and even economic reasons for not excluding people from access to drugs because of their inability to pay) had an obvious and instrumental role in the genesis of the pro-access regime. However, while being doubtless part of the impetus for action, these framings did not lead to a fundamental undermining of the power of the IPR/trade regime over the political economy of drugs. A brief discussion of the activities of the pro-access regime in relation to price and innovation interventions follows.

Price interventions

Financing partnerships and foundations clearly seek to increase drug availability via the disbursement of money. Organisations such as GAVI and the Global Fund, as well as foundations such as the Gates Foundation, have poured huge resources into financing greater access to certain types of medications, effectively subsidising drug interventions for select diseases in chosen countries. In practice, the disease focus of the major GHPs means that financing is disproportionately targeted at medicines and health technologies directed at the 'big three' diseases (HIV/AIDS, TB and malaria), while GAVI targets vaccines for preventable diseases. Although agencies such as the Global Fund and GAVI are able to point to considerable success in increasing access, their activities – and the model they represent – have not been immune to criticism. Concerns about the sustainability of such financing have become acute in the context of the financial crisis, but these concerns also preceded it (Williams and Rushton 2011). Also, questions about accountability plague these actors, not least of all with respect to accountability to patient groups and recipient developing countries (Birn 2005). The distorting effect of massive injections of finance on local drug manufacturers and national health systems have also received attention, as have instances of corruption, waste, endemic local parallel markets and the involvement of cost-raising middlemen in supply chains (England 2008, Shiffman 2008). Although it has improved access to some medications, the huge increase in finance has not served to challenge or solve long-term dynamic problems associated with drug production and supply (Kapczynski 2009).

However, there are two positive outcomes in the financing function of the pro-access actors, which might hold long-term positive effects for access to medicines more widely. The first relates to the widespread use of generics by these programmes, and the effects this has had on competition and price, and also the development of the generic sector, particularly in India. The second is the establishment of UNITAID in 2006 as a redistributive financing mechanism for the purchase of ARVs, an initiative which holds the promise of wider, innovative sustainable resourcing of pro-access initiatives.

These agencies have not, however, merely provided the financing for the purchase of drugs at existing prices; they have also sought to lower drug prices in order to increase the benefit that their resources can produce. In doing so, they have been joined by a number of other 'access organisations' (Caines 2004) and UN/WHO joint programmes with firms, such as the Accelerating Access Initiative (AAI). These organisations and programmes have led to the development of a range of price-intervention strategies, including differential pricing, drug donation schemes, and pooled procurement and price negotiations, as well as an increase in the use of generics (Oxfam 2007, Waning *et al.* 2009, Youde 2011).

Differential (or tiered) pricing schemes are in essence specific responses by pharmaceutical firms to differentiated pharmaceutical markets, often in regard to particularly morally and politically charged cases. The best example is the AAI, a partnership of nine pharmaceutical firms and five UN bodies, established in 2000 and directed to bringing down the price of ARTs. Both the AAI specifically and other firm-driven differential-pricing strategies have received criticism from a number of sources (Danzon and Towse 2003, Oxfam 2007), mainly over their dependence on the sustained commitment of firms, which has not always been steadfast. A recent, influential study by Waning *et al.* (2009) has also highlighted the fact that a price reduction gained by the generic entry of ARTs dwarfs those sustained by differentially priced equivalents. Differential prices can also have the function of short-term discounting to prevent the completion of entrance or to secure market dominance of a particular drug.

Donation programmes are perhaps the most extreme form of price reduction, effectively lowering the cost of the drugs involved to zero. Donation programmes to date have been restricted to some high-profile examples: Pfizer's Diflucan donation, Merck's Mectizan donation, the Boehringer donation of Viramune and so on. These programmes are managed by a corps of partners, charities and NGOs. However, such programmes have also had their critics, notably because of their effects on generic producers, the particular suitability of drugs or their relative efficacy, and the effect on the choice of treatment available to public-health bodies (WHO 1999). In particular, Ecks (2008) has traced how, as in the case of the Novartis donation scheme for Gilvec in India, the reasons behind donation schemes often reflect corporate strategy, not least of all to undercut generic competition, or to 'disguise' the fact that the markets in which prices can be cut are not the key ones at stake. Of course, for Ecks lower-priced or donated drugs in Southern markets serve to legitimise higher inflated prices in the core, lucrative markets that lie in the North (2008). But such programmes also chime well with corporate social responsibility, generate good PR and do not often represent balance sheet–busting donations of drugs with high market value. The Gilvec case is an important exception to this rule.

Pooled procurement is mainly undertaken by clusters of states or organisations seeking to purchase high volumes of a particular drug. Examples include consolidated drug-purchasing schemes managed by Pan American Health Organization (PAHO) or the vaccine-purchasing strategy of UNICEF, which is responsible for a 40% share of the total global vaccine market. In terms of partnerships, some successes have been witnessed under the Stop TB Partnership Global Drug Facility as well as the WHO's intervention in the artemisinin supply crisis, leading to huge reductions in price and increased volumes of global availability of artemisinin and ACTs. More recently, the Global Fund has established its own coordinating function – a scheme called Voluntary Pooled Procurement – with respect to block purchasing of ARTs (Kazatchkine *et al.* 2009). While this system has not yet had time to become established, Waning *et al.* (2009) note its potential to profoundly restructure the global ART market.

The negotiated price strategies pursued by the Clinton Foundation are in some ways linked to these high-volume/low-price strategies (Youde 2011). While largely confined to relations with generic ART producers (but increasingly active in anti-malarials and vaccines), the Clinton Foundation prides itself on taking a business approach to the problem of price. The foundation uses a series of techniques – such as demand forecasting – to lower the uncertainties involved for generic firms in matching investments in reverse engineering and production runs on the one hand, with predictable market size and sales volumes on the other (Youde 2011). The Clinton Foundation thus seeks to correct imperfect information (asymmetries) endemic to the ART markets, thereby lowering uncertainties as the basis for lower prices. Again, these strategies have scored some important successes in lowering prices, and the Clinton approach could hold real promise in reducing deadweight losses to consumers and producers as it is applied to other disease areas.

However, a number of more general problems for access to medicines are apparent from the price interventions of the pro-access regime. The first simply relates to the need for continued financing, or for intervention in the form of bargaining using obvious political clout in order to keep prices low. Often these interventions offer only short-term price reductions to patients who have a long-term need for treatment (as with ARTs). Problems will recur if either the money or the will to negotiate disappears. Second, it is clear that in most cases the entrance of generic production (especially in ARTs and ACTs) has had a dramatic impact on price, but that impact is only really systemic for a select few diseases. In many senses, this situation reflects the success of the human rights and public goods reframing of ARTs specifically within the post-2001 (Doha Declaration) IPR/trade regime. Since then, the question of ART compulsory licensing has largely proven to be 'exceptional', both with respect to corporations (and developed states) turning a blind eye to the enforcement of patent rights, and to the willingness of developing countries to enact compulsory licenses on them. As countries such as India (accounting for 80% of the global ARV generic supply) have acceded to TRIPS in 2005, and as TRIPS-plus agreements (including a currently negotiated EU–India FTA) ratchet up global IPRs, it is possible that price interventions based on generic entry into the global ART market – the change which has brought about by far the biggest reduction in prices – might prove to be only a temporary and 'exceptional' mechanism in terms of wider access. Other diseases and pro-access strategies will have to factor in higher prices to subsidise and longer durations to wait before generic competition permits the type of business-orientated, innovative solutions offered by the Clinton Foundation and others.

Innovation interventions

R&D and Product Development Partnerships (PDPs) are fairly straightforward to understand with respect to access to medicines; they bring together public and private medical research capabilities to provide the basis for innovation in neglected and other diseases. They thus correct market failure with respect to innovation. Their innovation-incentive function falls into two categories of activities: those organisations that supply push incentives (Kremer and Glennerster 2004) to the input side of R&D, and those that provide pull mechanisms – or offer alternate incentives for R&D and product development (Hecht *et al.* 2009).

Push mechanisms often take the form of financing of research efforts comprising both public and private bodies. Organisations such as the Gates Foundation, national governments and advocacy organisations (especially Rockefeller) have played pivotal roles in both the financial inputs and partnership brokerage necessary for PDPs to work. PDPs mostly rely on push incentives – often in the form of grants – and include actors such as the following: International AIDS Vaccine Initiative (IAVI), the Drugs for Neglected Diseases Initiative, the Malaria Vaccines Initiative, the Global Alliance for TB Drug Development and the Medicines for Malaria Venture. The Program for Appropriate Technology for Health (or PATH) receives approximately 63% of its budget from foundation sources, with the Gates Foundation injecting a massive $1.3 billion into its work on vaccines (and crop research) in 2009 (McCoy *et al.* 2009). These actors are clearly important when missing markets are a problem, with Moran *et al.* (2005) finding that PDPs accounted for three-quarters of all neglected-disease R&D projects, and others (Moran *et al.* 2007) noting considerable success in product development, with a staggering increase in the development of malaria vaccines being an exemplar. Similar R&D gains are reported by IAVI on trial candidates for HIV vaccines (Moran *et al.* 2007), with capacity building in developing countries (e.g. in laboratory personnel) being a real, positive externality of its R&D focus (Chattaway *et al.* 2009).

In an alternative approach to stimulating R&D, UNITAID has created a structure under which pharmaceutical companies can voluntarily contribute patents on ARVs. This allows others to research combination therapies in cases where patent rights and patent thickets otherwise present an obstacle (UNITAID 2007). The push element here derives from removing the considerable transaction, legal and financial costs that cross-licensing of multiple patents would otherwise involve, and thus eliminating a principal knock-on problem of patents. In 2010, the Medicines Patent Pool Foundation was established to administer the pool. Despite this positive initiative, it is clear that patent pools require financing and the largesse of the donating firms if they are to succeed.

Pull mechanisms are less evident in global health to date, although proposals for incentive structures to replicate the systemic function of IPRs are now legion. The most high profile of these ideas are those centring on the Health Impact Fund (HIF) and prizes (Hollis 2004, Hubbard and Love 2004, Pogge 2009). The basic idea of such schemes is to reward inventive activity in health by means of the impact of a new medicine on the global disease burden. The intention is to decouple innovation from price and patents while still supplying an incentive structure. Such systems and proposals have been intrinsically economically framed, both in terms of their critique of inefficiencies engendered by the patent system and in identification of the essentially short-term nature of some of the static interventions on innovation present in the push mechanisms described above. However, to date global health has only generated one significant pull mechanism, in the form of the Advanced Market Commitment that was established in 2007 using developed country, World Bank and Gates Foundation finances to secure a market (and guarantee a volume of sales) for a pneumococcal vaccine (Barder *et al.* 2006).

Part of the problem with push and pull mechanisms to date is that they fail to offer a systemic and stable means of generating innovation (Hollis 2004, Hubbard and Love 2004, Selgelid 2008). This is exactly the systemic incentive structure that profits and patents *do* supply, albeit, with unpalatable effects for access to medicines. The IPR/trade regime is also financially stable (in that it is underwritten largely by political will and higher consumer-end drug prices), and it is not dependent on foundation or state donations (Ravvin 2008). Push mechanisms can also introduce inefficiencies associated with the award of grants to the input end of R&D (Hollis and Pogge 2010), a stage at which successful end products are never guaranteed. Decisions about who gets the grants and which product lines to pursue can also be subject to bias and other problems associated with front-loading decisions about R&D (Hollis 2005, Ravvin 2008). Grant seeking by grant-dependent consortia can also further distort R&D and lead to waste.

The criticisms of these activities are not presented here in order to discount or undermine the successes of the price and innovation interventions developed by the pro-access regime. However, in the main these initiatives are piecemeal, disease-by-disease, and static responses to long-term and systemic economic problems of access to medicines. Only the HIF and prizes proposals show real merit as an economically efficient and practicable incentive system. Yet at present, the plans for a global HIF or alternatives remain only that – plans – and the transition to a parallel or replacement global system of access to medicines governance will require significant financing to constitute a level of rewards similar to that currently conferred by monopoly prices.

Conclusion

The obvious questions arising from this discussion concern how these two regimes (inter)relate with regard to access to medicines, and what the positive and negative consequences are of their attempts to respond to the particular problems of pharmaceutical production and innovation. Moreover, what does the evolution of governance responses to the issue tell us about social contestation and the uses of framing in the formation of global health policy?

First, in relation to the interaction of the two regimes examined here, a wider critical assessment suggests some limited grounds for optimism. It is clear that at the time of the Doha Declaration in 2001, the IPR/trade regime was facing a crisis with respect to the legitimacy of global drug patents. Sustained opposition by a sophisticated coalition of states, NGOs and HIV/AIDS activists promoted a substantial reframing, recasting the issue at stake in terms of development, human rights and public goods, rather than private rights. This produced a new policy momentum that coalesced around the select health interventions targeted by the MDGs, which were framed as (economic) development-orientated 'investments' in health, and especially HIV/AIDS. The disease-specific approach and pro-access interventions of the new actors that were born as a consequence of this new policy momentum have led to the huge expansion of coverage of select diseases (most especially HIV and malaria).

Yet, arguably, this pro-access regime has given new impetus and legitimacy to the IPR/trade regime and has helped to resolve its internal crisis by smoothing some of the rougher edges of its impact on access to medicines, particularly in the most politically charged case of access to ARTs. The pro-access regime has served this function (by design or by accident) as a result of its failure to substantially challenge the discourse that presents drug patenting as necessary for innovation, or to problematise the basic political economy of global pharmaceutical production and markets. Business here is very much as usual. While gains *have* been made in access, the vocal opposition to TRIPS and associated regimes, which was present in the period from 1996 to 2001, is no longer as forceful as it was. As that opposition has receded, the IPR/trade regime has reinvigorated itself by shifting the forums through which strong patents on medicines could be achieved (for example, in bilateral FTAs and new initiatives on piracy and counterfeiting), while continuing to frame the (economic) necessity of patents on drugs in strikingly similar ways to those used to justify TRIPS over two decades ago. Levels of protection are being 'ratcheted-up' at a time when political and financial commitment to even the big three diseases appears to be under siege.

However, in a more positive series of developments, it is clear that the pro-access regime is beginning to develop (at least in theory) a genuine and creative basis for incentivising drug innovation, most clearly in the area of neglected diseases. Many of the PDPs, prize funds and other push and pull mechanisms are reliant on continued donor funds, but there are also signals indicating that new redistributive sources of financing might allow for a sustainable parallel system of incentives to fund new drug discovery (as in the case of UNITAID). If these types of approaches were expanded, they could offer a route out of the economic problems that currently plague access to medicines.

Finally, with regard to the contested framing of access to medicines, it is worth noting that the economic framing or justification of the IPR/trade regime has proven particularly resilient. From the mid-1990s (and even up to the present), the IPR/trade regime was 'successfully' counter-framed in terms of its negative human rights consequences for access to medicines, its undermining of global public goods and its negative impact on international development. Despite legal victories for access-to-medicines campaigners within the WTO-TRIPS and other arenas, new platforms, forums and levels of governance have been deployed to strengthen the wider IPR/trade regime. However, now a growing body of literature and policy initiatives (such as HIF, PDPs and even UNITAID) are increasingly challenging the basic assumptions of the economic case for both global and national drug patents, focusing on their negative impact on rates of innovation and price. Indeed, these quintessentially economic critiques are increasingly emerging from actors and individuals closely associated with the first wave of human rights and development counter-framings of the IPR/trade regime. The arguments that have been used by proponents of strong drug patents are now being challenged on their own (economic) grounds, highlighting the fact that those arguments are often internally inconsistent, dysfunctional and deeply flawed with regard to innovation and access to medicines. New policies and governance arrangements have only recently responded to the economic problems associated with this dysfunctional system. While there are promising signs of genuine change, these developments operate only in the margins of an IPR/trade regime, which remains the only truly systemic form of governance in the access to medicines area.

Acknowledgements

This research has been made possible through funding from the European Research Council under the European Community's Seventh Framework Programme – Ideas Grant 230489 GHG. All views expressed remain those of the authors.

Note

1. A perspective borne out by extensive interviews conducted with UN and other organisation personnel as part of the European Research Council (ERC) project.

References

Abbott, F.M., 2002. The TRIPS agreement, access to medicines and the Doha Ministerial Conference. *The journal of world intellectual property*, 5 (1), 15–52.

Baker, D., 2004. Financing drug research: what are the issues? 2008 Industry Studies Conference paper. Available from: http://ssrn.com/abstract=1134983 [Accessed 1 Aug 2011].

Barder, O., Kremer, M., and Williams, H., 2006. Advanced market commitments: a policy to stimulate investment in vaccines and neglected diseases. *Economists' voice*, 1–5 Feb, pp. 1–6.

Barton, J.H. and Emanuel, E.J., 2005. The patents-based pharmaceutical development process: rationale, problems, and potential reform. *Journal of the American medical association*, 294 (16), 2075–2082.

Birn, A.-E., 2005. Gate's grandest challenge: transcending technology as a public health ideology. *The Lancet*, 366 (9484), 514–519.

Black, R.E., Bhan, M., Chopra, M., Rudan, I., and Victoria, C., 2009. Accelerating the health impact of the Gates Foundation. *The Lancet*, 373 (9675), 1584–1585.

Braga, C.A.P., 1989. Economics of intellectual property rights and the GATT: a view from the South. *Vanderbilt journal of transnational law*, 22, 243–264.

Braga, C.A.P., Fink, C., and Sepulveda, C.P., 2000. *Intellectual property rights and economic development*. World Bank discussion paper, number 412, Washington DC: World Bank.

Caines, K., 2004. *Global health partnerships and neglected diseases*. London: DFID Health Resource Centre.

Chattaway, J., Hanlin, R., Mugwagwa, J., and Muraguri, I., 2009. Global health social technologies: reflections on evolving theories and landscapes. Innogen Working Paper, 76. Available from: http://oro.open.ac.uk/29783 [Accessed 14 Dec 2011].

Danzon, P. and Towse, A., 2003. Differential pricing for pharmaceuticals: reconciling access, R&D and patents. *International journal of health care finance and economics*, 3, 183–205.

Drahos, P., 2003. Expanding intellectual property's empire: the role of FTAs. Available from: http://ictsd.net/downloads/2008/08/drahos-fta-2003-en.pdf [Accessed 11 Aug 2011].

Drahos, P. and Braithwaite, J., 2002. *Information feudalism: who owns the knowledge economy?* London: Earthscan Press.

Ecks, S., 2008. Global pharmaceutical markets and corporate citizenship: the case of Novartis' anti-cancer drug Glivec. *BioSocieties*, 3 (2), 165–181.

England, R., 2008. The writing is on the wall for UNAIDS. *British medical journal*, 336 (7652), 1072.

Faunce, T.A. and Lexchin, J., 2007. 'Linkage' pharmaceutical evergreening in Australia and Canada. *Australia and New Zealand health policy*, 4 (8), 1–11.

Flynn, S., Hollis, A., and Palmedo, M., 2009. An economic justification for open access to essential medicine patents in developing countries. *The Journal of law and medicine*, 37 (2), 184–208.

Grabowski, H., 2002. Patents, innovation and access to new pharmaceuticals. *Journal of international economic law*, 5 (4), 849–860.

Hecht, R., Wilson, P., and Palriwala, A., 2009. Improving health R&D financing for developing countries: a menu of innovative policy options. *Health affairs*, 28 (4), 974–985.

Helfer, L.R., 2004. Regime shifting: the TRIPS agreement and new dynamics of international intellectual property law making. *Yale journal of international law*, 29 (1), 1–83.

Hollis A., 2005. An efficient reward system for pharmaceutical innovation. Available from: http://www.who.int/intellectualproperty/news/en/Submission-Hollis.pdf [Accessed 10 Aug 2011].

Hollis, A. and Pogge, T., 2010. The Health Impact Fund: making new medicines accessible for all. Incentives for Global Health. Available from: http://www.healthimpactfund.org [Accessed 5 Aug 2011].

Hubbard, T. and Love, J., 2004 A new trade framework for global healthcare R&D. *PLoS Biology*, 2 (2), e52. doi: 10.1371/journal.pbio.0020052.

Johnston, J. and Wasunna, A., 2007. Patents, biomedical research and treatments: examining concerns, canvassing solutions. *Hastings center report*, 37, S1–S36.

Kapczynski, A., 2009. Harmonization and its discontents: a case study of TRIPS implementation in India's pharmaceutical sector. *California law review*, 97, 1571–1649.

Kazatchkine, M.D., Atun, R., and Lansang, M.-A., 2009. Global health partnerships: a 'pull' mechanism for innovation and new products. *Global forum update on research for health*, 6, 138–141.

Kinsella, N.S., 2001. Against intellectual property. *Journal of libertarian studies*, 15 (2), 1–53.

Kremer, M., 2002. Pharmaceuticals and the developing world. *Journal of economic perspectives*, 16 (4), 67–90.

Kremer, M. and Glennerster, R., 2004. *Strong medicine: creating incentives for pharmaceutical research on neglected diseases*. Princeton, NJ: Princeton University Press.

Lanjouw, J.O., 1998. *The introduction of product pharmaceutical patents in India*. "Heartless exploitation of the poor and suffering" NBER Working Paper No. 6366. Available from: http://www.nber.org/papers/w6366.pdf?new_window=1 [Accessed 1 Sept 2011].

Mansfield, E., 1986. Patents and innovation: an empirical study. *Management science*, 32 (2), 173–181.

McCoy, D., Kembhavi, G., Patel, J., and Luintel, A., 2009. The Bill and Melinda Gates Foundation's grant-making programme for global health. *The Lancet*, 373 (9675), 1645–1653.

Moran, M., Ropars, A.-L., Guzman, J., Diaz, J., and Garrison, C., 2005. *The new landscape of neglected disease drug development*. London: LSE/Wellcome Trust.

Moran, M., Ropars, A.-L., Guzman, J., Jorgensen, M., McDonald, A., Potter, S., and Salassie, H.H., 2007. *The malaria product pipeline; planning for the future*. Sydney: Health Policy Division, George Institute for International Health.

Muzaka, V., 2010. Linkages, contests and overlaps in the global intellectual property rights regime. *European journal of international relations*, 20 (10), 1–22.

Odell, J.S. and Sell, S.K., 2006. Reframing the issue: the WTO coalition on intellectual property and public health, 2001. *In*: J.S. Odell, ed. *Negotiating trade: Developing countries in the WTO and NAFTA*. Cambridge: Cambridge University Press, 85–113.

Oxfam. 2007. *Investing for life. Meeting poor people's needs for access to medicines through responsible business practices*. Oxford: Oxfam.

Pogge, T., 2009. The Health Impact Fund: boosting pharmaceutical innovation without obstructing free access. *Cambridge quarterly of healthcare ethics*, 18 (1), 78–86.

Ravishankar, N., Gubbins, P., Cooley, R.J., Leach-Kemon, K., Michaud, C.M., Jamison, D.T., and Murray, C.J.L., 2009. Financing of global health: tracking development assistance for health from 1990 to 2007. *The Lancet*, 373 (9681), 2113–2124.

Ravvin, M., 2008. Incentivizing access and innovation for essential medicines: a survey of the problem and proposed solutions. *Public health ethics*, 2 (1), 110–123.

Rosiello, A. and Smith, J., 2004. A sociological economy of HIV(AIDS vaccine partnerships: case studies from Africa and India. *International review of sociology*, 18 (2), 283–299.

Rushton, S. and Williams, O.D., eds., 2011. *Partnerships and foundations in global health governance*. Basingstoke: Palgrave.

Selgelid, M.J., 2008. A full-pull program for the provision of pharmaceuticals: practical issues. *Public health ethics*, 1 (2), 134–145.

Sell, S.K., 2002. TRIPS and the access to medicines campaign. *Wisconsin international law journal*, 20 (3), 481–522.

Sell, S.K. and Prakash, A., 2004. Using ideas strategically: the contest between business and NGO networks in intellectual property rights. *International studies quarterly*, 48 (1), 143–175.

Shiffman, J., 2008. Has donor prioritization of HIV(AIDS displaced aid for other health issues? *Health policy and planning*, 23 (2), 95–100.

Stiglitz, J.E., 2007. Prizes, not patents. *Project Syndicate*. Available from: http://www.project-syndicate.org/commentary/stiglitz81/English [Accessed 19 Jul 2011].

Stiglitz, J.E., 1999. Knowledge as a global public good. *In*: I. Kaul, I. Grunberg, and M.A. Stern, eds. *Global public goods*. New York: Oxford University Press, 308–328.

Stiglitz, J.E., 2008. Economic foundations of intellectual property rights. *Duke law journal*, 57, 1693–723.

Trouiller, P., Olliaro, P., Torreele, E., Orbinski, J., Laing, R., and Ford, N., 2002. Drug development for neglected diseases: a deficient market and a public-health policy failure. *The Lancet*, 359 (9324), 2188–2194.

UNAIDS. 2012. *Together we will end AIDS*. Available from: http://www.unaids.org/en/media/unaids/contentassets/documents/epidemiology/2012/20120718_togetherwewillendaids_en.pdf [Accessed 5 Jul 2012].

UNITAID. 2007. *UNITAID Mission*. Available from: http://www.unitaid.eu/index.php/en/UNITAID-Mission.html [Accessed 23 Mar 2011].

UN Millennium Project. 2005. *Prescription for healthy development: increasing access to essential medicines*. Report of the Taskforce on HIV/AIDS, Malaria, TB, and Access to Medicines, Working Group on Access to Essential Medicines. Sterling, VA: Earthscan.

Waning, B., Kaplan, W., King, A.C., Lawrence, D.A., Luefkens, H.G., and Fox, M.P., 2009. Global strategies to reduce the price of antiretroviral medicines: evidence from transactional databases. *Bulletin of the world health organization*, 87, 520–528.

WHO, 1999. *Guidelines for drug donations*. Geneva: WHO. Available from: http://apps.who.int/medicinedocs/en/d/Jwhozip52e [Accessed 14 Dec 2011].

Williams, O.D. and Rushton, S., 2011. Are the 'good times' over? Looking to the future of Global Health Governance. *Global health governance*, 5 (1), 1–16.

Woodling, M., Williams, O.D., and Rushton, S., 2012. New life in old frames: HIV, development and the 'AIDS plus MDGs' approach. *Global public health*, 7 (10), Supplement 3 (this volume).

WTO. 1994. Agreement on trade related aspects of intellectual property rights, Marrakesh Agreement establishing the World Trade Organization, Annex 1C, Legal instruments-results of the Uruguay round, 1869 U.N.T.S. 299, 33 J.L.M. 1197.

WTO. 2001. *Doha Declaration on TRIPS and public health*. Geneva: WTO. Available from: http://www.wto.org/english/thewto_e/minist_e/min01_e/mindecl_trips_e.htm [Accessed 14 Dec 2011].

Youde, J., 2011. The Clinton Foundation and Global Health Governance. *In*: S. Rushton and O.D. Williams, eds. *Partnerships and foundations in Global Health Governance*. Basingstoke: Palgrave, 164–181.

New life in old frames: HIV, development and the 'AIDS plus MDGs' approach

Marie Woodling, Owain D. Williams and Simon Rushton

Centre for Health and International Relations (CHAIR), Department of International Politics, Aberystwyth University, Aberystwyth, UK

There have been recent indications that the primacy of AIDS among global health issues may be under threat. In this article we examine one response to have emerged from the AIDS policy community as a result of this perceived threat: the 'AIDS plus Millennium Development Goals (MDGs)' approach, which argues that the AIDS response (the focus of MDG6) is essential to achieving the other MDG targets by 2015, stressing the two-way relationship between AIDS and other development issues. By framing AIDS in this way, the AIDS plus MDGs approach draws on an established narrative of a 'virtuous circle' between health and development, but at the same time makes some important concessions to critics of the AIDS response. This article – the first critical academic analysis of the AIDS plus MDGs approach – uses this case to illuminate aspects of the utilisation of framing in global health, shedding light both on the extent to which new framings draw upon established 'common sense' narratives as well as the ways in which framers must adapt to the changing material and ideational context in which they operate.

Introduction

AIDS has been the most prominent issue on the global health agenda in the 21st century. The global response to AIDS has involved substantial political will and the commitment of unprecedented resources, as well as the creation of new international institutions such as the Joint United Nations Programme on HIV/AIDS (UNAIDS) and funding platforms such as the Global Fund to Fight AIDS, TB and Malaria (the Global Fund). One of the explanations that has been put forward in the literature for this degree of prioritisation is that the AIDS policy community has been particularly successful at framing and reframing the pandemic at various times and in various ways to capture high-level political attention (Shiffman 2009, Rushton 2010). As Shiffman (2009, p. 609) notes, 'HIV/AIDS has been framed as a public health problem, a development issue, a humanitarian crisis, a human rights issue and a threat to security'.

One of the most prominent themes in the literature on AIDS, in international relations in particular, has been an examination of the 'securitisation' of AIDS – in other words, the way in which AIDS has been framed and constructed as a security issue (Elbe 2006, Prins 2004). Examples such as the UN Security Council's Resolution 1308 in 2000 on AIDS as a security issue and the influence of security considerations in motivating the US's major programme on AIDS – the President's Emergency Plan for AIDS Relief (PEPFAR) – have been used to exemplify the ways in which the security framing has played a part in mobilising political will and resources for AIDS (Ingram 2009). It is notable, however, that the rhetoric around AIDS as a security issue is far less prominent now than it was a decade ago (McInnes and Rushton 2010). Here, we focus on an alternative framing of AIDS as a development issue, which has been as significant in motivating international attention as security (if not more so) and remains prominent in the AIDS policy discourse. In particular, we examine how AIDS has recently been framed by two of the key global AIDS and development institutions, UNAIDS and the United Nations Development Programme (UNDP), through the policy initiative 'AIDS plus MDGs'. In this initiative, UNAIDS and UNDP are drawing on a long history of AIDS (and indeed health more broadly) being linked with international development, but are doing so in an instrumental way that is responsive to the prevailing economic and policy contexts both these actors and global health and development more generally presently face. What this reveals are a number of insights into the power of frames and the use of framing by actors in global health governance.

We begin by tracing the historical narrative that has established the central position of AIDS as a 'development problem', showing the ways in which this emerged from earlier debates on health and development, and became institutionalised through the MDGs, the Commission on Macroeconomics and Health (CMH) and other processes. In the second section we examine in detail two recent documents (published by UNAIDS and UNDP/UNAIDS, respectively) that draw upon this narrative to (re)frame AIDS as a development problem in a particular way. Although this AIDS plus MDGs approach represents only one of the initiatives currently being pursued by these agencies, the ways in which they seek to (re)frame AIDS are interesting and significant. The documents we examine were produced in a context in which AIDS has been criticised for receiving disproportionate prioritisation (as found in the debate over AIDS exceptionalism), in which other health priorities have increasingly been challenging AIDS' supremacy, and in which the global financial crisis has led to increased resource pressures on all areas of health and development. In response to this difficult environment, UNAIDS and UNDP have sought to strategically forward the case through the AIDS plus MDGs approach that AIDS is inextricably linked to the other MDG goals, and that the AIDS response should be taken out of isolation, yet still prioritised as a key to achieving the MDGs more broadly. In this sense, this example of the framing of AIDS clearly resonates with an established historical narrative about the existence of a 'virtuous circle' between AIDS and development (with AIDS interventions often being presented as the starting point for creating that positive relationship), yet operationalises that narrative in a new way for a particular political purpose. In the conclusion to the paper we seek to draw out the implications for our understanding of the use of framing in global health governance, in particular shedding light both on the extent to which new framings draw upon established narratives and also on the ways in which framers adapt their message to the changing material and ideation contexts in which they operate.

AIDS, poverty and development: establishing a narrative

In this section we briefly outline the historical process through which AIDS came to be widely viewed as one of the foremost international development challenges. We first examine the rise of international development as a high-level global policy priority, commanding real resources and backed by significant political will. The MDGs are a sign of this prioritisation, and the extent to which resources have been mobilised towards achieving them (in stark comparison with previous failed 'decades of development') is a clear illustration of development's new status. We then examine how AIDS (and to a lesser extent other select diseases) came to be privileged in relation to other health issues, and how a narrative became established that AIDS is one of the principal obstacles to development – a narrative which drew upon an older 'virtuous circle' argument that investing in health could have broader development benefits. Finally, in this section we address some of the critiques of AIDS' exceptional position and some of the pressures being faced by the AIDS community in recent years.

It is clear that there was, at the turn of the new millennium, a generally increased level of political concern with issues such as development, debt and the environment. This cannot be attributed to any single cause or event, but rather to a number of different sources of momentum which coalesced. For example, through the 1990s the issue of Third World debt was taken up as a popular cause, including high-profile celebrity interventions. This movement focused on advocating for debt relief/ forgiveness, and was most concretely expressed through the Jubilee 2000 campaign. Governments – particularly certain global leaders (including Tony Blair, Gordon Brown, Bill Clinton and Al Gore) – were also pivotal in championing a range of development issues, seen perhaps most clearly in a series of high-level summits (including the G8 meetings at Okinawa in 2000 and Gleneagles in 2005) that addressed core issues of international development and the challenges facing Africa as a continent. Crucially, the G8 support for development agendas, not least in health, supplied both the necessary political sanction for action and the promise of resources. Yet, in addition to this agency, context was also important, including the fact that the huge new investment in health and development occurred after a decade of global economic growth, and at a time of relative economic prosperity in the West.

The adoption of the MDGs in 2001 was perhaps the most high-profile and influential product of this zeitgeist. The MDGs do not, and were never intended to, address *all* development needs. It was always recognised that even achieving them would be only a first step towards economic development and that reaching the goals was not an end itself but part of a longer process. Nevertheless, over the first 15 years of the 21st century, the MDGs have been at the heart of the global development agenda. Not all current development activities are explicitly MDG-related, but many are. The various institutions of the UN, for example, have either formally or informally linked their programmes and activities to the MDG goals, as have many national development agencies such as the Department for International Development (DFID) in the UK. New institutions such as the Global Fund have been created specifically to address particular MDG targets. The MDGs, therefore, have been influential not only in setting the development agenda, but in shaping the very architecture of global development. The power of the goal- and target-setting function of the MDGs with respect to development should not be underestimated, and neither should the scale of resources from major donors invested in moving towards achieving them. Indeed, such has been the power of the MDGs in channelling global development efforts that many of the previous debates over what development *means* (debates that continue within academia and civil society) have been dramatically downplayed.

The recent (2011) Fourth High-Level Forum on Aid Effectiveness in Busan, South Korea, saw countries recommitting to the MDGs, highlighting the fact that the Millennium Declaration 'sets out our universal mandate for development' and stressing the need for new approaches that move beyond traditional modes of aid delivery in order to achieve them. Despite the financial crisis, therefore, the MDGs clearly remain an important touchstone in development and in international politics more widely. Other approaches and understandings of development persist and remain influential – see, for example, the 'capabilities approach' associated with Nussbaum and Sen (1993). But, as Ollila (2005) points out, the policy space for other approaches to both health and development has shrunk as a result of the dominance of the MDG agenda.

One of the major beneficiaries of the MDG target-setting process was AIDS which, along with malaria and 'other diseases' (among which TB has probably been the most prominent), formed the focus of MDG6. It is notable that MDG6 led directly to the creation of the Global Fund in 2002, which is one of the largest and most innovative new health-governance initiatives. There was, however, nothing natural or pre-ordained about the inclusion of AIDS in the MDGs. As David Hulme (2007) points out, AIDS had not been included in previously negotiated sets of targets. The Organisation for Economic Co-operation and Development-Development Assistance Committee's (OECD-DAC) International Development Goals (effectively the forerunner of the MDGs), for example, made no explicit mention of AIDS. Yet the General Assembly's Millennium Declaration (UN General Assembly 2000) pledged to have 'halted, and begun to reverse, the spread of HIV/AIDS, the scourge of malaria and other major diseases that afflict humanity' by 2015 – the target encapsulated in MDG6.

What the Millennium Declaration did not do, however, is set out clearly the reasons *why* the General Assembly considered AIDS to be a particular priority and worthy of a specific target. Self-evidently, the Millennium Declaration draws upon a framework rooted in development (and economic development in particular), although in various places the document also makes references to security and human rights. But if we examine the backstory to the Millennium Declaration, the way in which AIDS came to be framed as a key development challenge is more clearly evident. For this we need to look at *We the Peoples* (Annan 2000), former Secretary-General Kofi Annan's report to the General Assembly prior to the Millennium Summit, from which the final declaration was drawn. It was AIDS' inclusion in *We the Peoples* – which has been attributed to the personal view of Mr Annan and some of his close advisors (especially John Ruggie) that HIV/AIDS is a key obstacle to development (Traub 2006, pp. 147–170) – that ultimately led to its being highlighted in MDG6. Such is the emphasis on HIV/AIDS in that report that Hulme (2007, p. 10) notes that, 'a Martian reading the final chapter of *We the Peoples* could reasonably conclude that HIV/AIDS was the only health problem facing the Earth's poor people'. Other health issues (including low spending on health care; a lack of research into neglected diseases such as pneumonia, diarrhoea, tuberculosis and malaria; and a lack of access to drugs, vaccines and other basic interventions) *are* highlighted in the report. However, after briefly noting them, Mr Annan makes the following striking statement:

> It is beyond the scope of this report to explore all of these challenges. I wish here to focus on a specific health crisis that threatens to reverse a generation of accomplishments in human development, and which is rapidly becoming a social crisis on a global scale: the spread of HIV/AIDS. (Annan 2000)

This statement, and the discussion which follows it, is arguably *the* key move in terms of the prioritisation of AIDS via its explicit inclusion in the MDGs, and in reinforcing the link between AIDS and development.

This was certainly not, however, the first time in which health issues had been linked to economic development, and Mr Annan's statements on AIDS drew upon a well-established framing of health as an obstacle to development, and specifically economic development. A seminal moment in the establishment of this narrative was the World Bank's hugely influential 1993 World Development Report titled '*Investing in Health*'. Not only did the report focus exclusively on health, it suggested that poor health was a primary obstacle to development and thereby justified investment in health in terms of poverty alleviation, net economic return on investment and horizontal spill-overs of such investments to other areas of development. This was a game-changing rhetorical shift: a move away from viewing health as a *cost* governments face to seeing it instead as an *investment opportunity*. Crucial to this case was the idea of the potential for a virtuous circle between health spending, productivity and economic development. Investments in health were held to be cost-effective (as compared to other development stimuli) and justifiable in terms of the economic and social returns. The virtuous-circle narrative subsequently gained traction, coming to colonise the discourses of other high-profile development institutions, with the health-to-economic development linkage appearing increasingly natural and obvious. The UNDP's (1996) Human Development Report, for example, noted that: 'Human development requires, among other things, considerable investment in education, health and nutrition. The result is a healthier and better educated population that is capable of being economically more productive' (p. 66).

While the MDGs rest implicitly upon the virtuous-circle idea that investing in health (and other key areas) can help kick-start economic growth in developing countries, that argument was set out even more clearly in the 2001 report of the WHO-backed CMH, under the chairmanship of Jeffrey Sachs. The report represented a natural and conscious counterpart to the MDGs themselves, but crucially it economically justified the selection of specific – or 'select disease' – interventions in global health (for example, investing in combating specific diseases) in the name of poverty elimination and development. This added to the economic justifications for the vertical disease-specific approach embodied in MDG6 in particular. It also reinforced the disease-focused nature of global health policy-making and the privileging of disease-specific interventions over wider (horizontal) systems-focused approaches to health and poverty, not to mention investments in things such as sanitation and clean drinking water, which have been recognised as playing a long-term, dramatic role in improving population health.

The CMH's report also shared a common approach with earlier framings of health as a target of investment that can lead to improvements in economic productivity and economic development more generally, while also presenting poor health as an obstacle to development: in short the vicious/virtuous-circle argument. For critics such as Alison Katz, however, this 'common sense' assumption – evident in both the 1993 World Bank Report and the 2001 CMH Report – is deeply problematic. For one, she argues the following:

> The relationship between health and poverty is two way but it is *not symmetric.* Poverty is the single most important determinant of poor health. But poor health is very far from being the single most important determinant of poverty. Poor health exacerbates existing poverty. Both the vicious cycle and the "virtuous" cycle of health and poverty are misleading images, as they imply equal weight of the two poles of health and economic development. (Katz 2004, p. 752)

Secondly, Katz highlights the existence of alternative and arguably more significant determinants of poverty in developing countries than health. These include the skewed international terms of trade (2005, pp. 179–180); the burden of developing country debt as compared to aid receipts and the failure of the Highly Indebted Poor Countries initiative (HIPO) (p. 179); and western intervention (both military and economic) in such countries (p. 182). Thus, she argues, poor health should be viewed as *only one* outcome of, rather than the principal driver of, these wider relations and structures (p. 176). Also, while investing in health will benefit the populations of developing countries, it will not succeed in fundamentally addressing the problems of poverty and underdevelopment unless some of the other (and more powerful) root causes are also addressed. Whether one agrees with Katz's critique or not, it is clear from the examples examined here that the vicious/virtuous circle argument has become deeply entrenched within current thinking on the relationship between health and development.

Among the 'select diseases' that have dominated 21st century global health, AIDS has been by far the most prominent and the biggest recipient of investment. The MDGs placed AIDS in a privileged position vis-à-vis other global health issues and even other select diseases. Although the MDGs set out measurable targets in respect to three health issues: infant mortality (MDG4); maternal mortality (MDG5); and HIV/AIDS, malaria and 'other diseases' (MDG6), of these three so-called 'health MDGs' it is clear that HIV/AIDS has received by far the most sustained focus and has captured a huge proportion of the global health expenditure (notwithstanding a renewed vigour in the area of childhood vaccination, reflected in the 2011 refinancing of GAVI), often at the expense of the 'competing' health MDGs (not to mention those health issues not covered by the MDGs).

One of the results of this focus on AIDS in the MDGs has been the transposition of the broader 'common sense' narrative of health-to-development to a new common sense narrative of AIDS-to-development, despite evidence that the causal relation-ship between poverty and AIDS is far more complex. It is not simply the case that being poor makes you more likely to contract HIV (Gould 2009), nor that AIDS is the principal driver of global poverty. Nevertheless, investing heavily in AIDS has come to be a central pillar of international development efforts, and these background assumptions that investing in HIV/AIDS prevention, treatment and care helps to address one of the most significant obstacles to development are never far from the surface.

More recently, however, the privileged status of AIDS and its 'exceptional' status with regard to development spending have come under challenge, partly as a result of the success in capturing funding and concerns over the distorting effects of that success on other areas. For example, Shiffman (2008) traces how international aid for HIV/AIDS has had a number of distorting effects on other areas of health aid and development, claiming that this has led to some loss of focus on other key global health challenges, including stagnation in funding for strengthening health systems. Roger England (2008, p. 1072), on the other hand, takes a more radical approach. He highlights that while AIDS accounts for 3.7% of global mortality, 'it receives 25% of international healthcare aid', a fact which he sees as distorting international health funding; as out of proportion; as having the potential to cause disruption to (fragile) national health systems; and as a reason for immediate institutional reform in the shape of dismantling UNAIDS.

The AIDS community and the major AIDS institutions are responding to these challenges – as well as to other pressures generated by the financial crisis and the perception of shifting donor priorities (especially towards maternal health and malaria). This has included a concerted attempt to provide a justification for AIDS' ongoing prioritisation. In the next section we examine one of the ways in which two of these institutions have sought to present this argument: the AIDS plus MDGs approach. Clearly, the institutions involved (UNAIDS and UNDP) have simultaneously been involved in other policy initiatives, including high-profile strategies such as 'Getting to Zero' which has been a prominent part of UNAIDS' recent position on the future of AIDS financing. Notwithstanding these other initiatives, the AIDS plus MDGs approach is interesting in that it seeks to reposition AIDS in a way that mobilises the established virtuous-circle arguments, but both repackages them for the contemporary policy context (in which there is a major emphasis on the MDG deadline of 2015) and makes some significant concessions to the critics of 'silo-based' global health strategies and AIDS exceptionalism.

The AIDS plus MDGs approach

The AIDS plus MDGs approach has to date been driven by UNAIDS and UNDP, with discussion on the approach beginning at the UNAIDS Committee of Cosponsoring Organizations in 2009 (UNDP/UNAIDS 2011, p. 23). The concept became a more prominent feature of international discussions in 2010, and was a particular focus for UNAIDS at the May 2010 World Health Assembly and the September 2010 MDG Review Summit. At the latter event, there was a widespread perception that other health issues, not least maternal health and malaria, were beginning to threaten AIDS' dominance of the policy agenda. During the summit, UNAIDS and the governments of China, South Africa and Nigeria co-hosted a side event on the AIDS plus MDGs approach that included keynote speakers from a number of heavily affected countries as well as WHO Director-General Margaret Chan and Michel Sidibé, Executive Director of UNAIDS (UNAIDS 2010a). UNAIDS has subsequently continued to promote the AIDS plus MDGs approach.

The AIDS plus MDGs approach highlights the intersections between AIDS (the focus of MDG6) and the other MDG targets, making the following case:

AIDS and the other MDGs are fundamentally interrelated. An effective AIDS response is critical to the achievement of the other MDGs, particularly in high-prevalence areas. Conversely, making a substantial impact on the AIDS pandemic depends on simultaneously advancing progress in other MDG areas. (Kim *et al.* 2011, p. 144)

The crux of the argument is that an approach to AIDS that views it within the context of the MDGs as a whole would provide 'an opportunity to respond in a fresh way to the changing context and to accelerate progress in achieving the MDGs' (UNAIDS 2010b, p. 3). Rather than stressing only the positive effects on other areas of development through investing in AIDS, the approach examined here supplements this with a more sensitive view of the positive effects on AIDS as a result of investment in other MDG areas (such as education, maternal health and poverty alleviation). In addition, this approach acknowledges the wider structural determinants of HIV and health status. The agenda forwarded by the AIDS plus MDGs approach therefore presents itself as a recontextualisation of AIDS' place within development and reframes the AIDS–development relationship in more bidirectional and interdependent terms. AIDS is still cast as one of the major obstacles to development, yet structural factors associated with underdevelopment are also included in the frame as obstacles to real progress on AIDS.

This shift in thinking can be seen as a response to a number of changes in the political and economic environment within which global AIDS and health institutions now find themselves. First, as Whiteside (2009) has indicated, the period from 2006 onwards has witnessed an unprecedented challenge to AIDS exceptionalism with regard to development policy and aid. Debates surrounding the distorting role of AIDS on overall health and development spending; the desirability of shifting investment to health systems and Health Systems Strengthening; concerns about the absorptive capacity of countries; a growing belief that the global AIDS response may be reaching the limits of what can be achieved without taking a broader approach; and changing ideas about the nature of a 'sustainable' global response have all played a part in generating new thinking and changing priorities. The AIDS plus MDGs approach also explicitly seeks to address the changing economic context of international development, not least the impact of the global financial crisis and apparent changes in political prioritisation. Thus the AIDS plus MDGs approach should properly be viewed as an attempt to provide a response to many of these criticisms and problems (which have come from both within and outside the AIDS policy community), but it does so in a manner that seeks to limit the damage to AIDS' status as a top-tier health and development issue and provides an adjusted rationale for continued (and indeed increased) investment in AIDS.

The remainder of this section provides an analysis of two of the key policy documents laying out the AIDS plus MDGs approach, presenting evidence of both continuity and change vis-à-vis previous framings of health, AIDS and development. The first is a UNAIDS document titled 'AIDS plus MDGs: synergies that serve people' (UNAIDS 2010b). The second is a 2011 UNDP/UNAIDS publication titled 'The "AIDS and MDGs" approach: what is it, why does it matter, and how do we take it forward?' (UNDP/UNAIDS 2011). A version of the latter paper authored by members of the UNDP's HIV/AIDS Group was also published in the journal *Third World Quarterly* (Kim *et al.* 2011). The two documents clearly overlap, and both draw on the same well-established discourses that link AIDS, poverty and development in the notion of the virtuous circle. However, both documents also show strategic adjustment to changing circumstances and policy critiques that accrued during the first decade of the MDG period.

The clearest areas of continuity lie in the documents' depiction of AIDS as being fundamentally linked to development. Both documents place a considerable emphasis upon the structural determinants of HIV and the need for HIV and development policy to be viewed holistically. For example, the UNAIDS document argues the following:

> To be effective and sustainable, the AIDS response, working strategically with other development partners, must continue and ramp up its push for positive social change and become more holistic in approaching these drivers and the companion health, development and rights challenges that affect and are affected by the epidemic—like maternal and child health, gender violence and inequality, universal education and infectious diseases like tuberculosis. AIDS responses must reach beyond the artificial boundaries of a single disease. (UNAIDS 2010b, p. 3)

However, little attempt is made in the documents to explain what is meant by 'development', other than a focus on the other MDGs. Perhaps this focus on the MDGs is natural enough since, as we noted above, the MDGs have formed a blueprint for health and development policy for the last decade, but again we find that the AIDS plus MDGs approach collapses this broader (and highly contested) development paradigm into a narrow focus on MDG attainment. Obviously, this evades the complexity of defining development and clarifying the various dimensions of its relationship with HIV/AIDS and obscures the highly politicised terrain which the relationship has traditionally occupied. However, as is often the case with the use of a contested concept, the use of development nonetheless introduces a tension. While the AIDS plus MDGs approach embodies in theory a clear recognition of the myriad links between HIV and development more broadly, these documents were both written within a policy context defined by – and therefore naturally focusing upon – the eight internationally agreed MDG goals rather than a more comprehensive understanding of development.

Also evident throughout the documents is the well-established claim that investing in AIDS has spill-over effects for other MDGs, creating a virtuous circle in which both AIDS and other development problems are addressed: 'An effective AIDS response is critical to the achievement of the other MDGs, particularly in high prevalence areas' (UNDP/UNAIDS 2011, p. 9). This general argument is supplemented in both documents through the use of case studies to show the broader impacts of AIDS investments in practice in countries such as Rwanda, Ethiopia and Nigeria. Both documents also provide examples of a number of ways in which HIV investments benefit the other MDG targets. The UNDP/UNAIDS document in particular provides a wealth of evidence of this impact on a number of the other MDGs (2011, p. 21), in each case providing references to studies that provide evidence of the link. This cross-cutting role of AIDS is also strongly in evidence in the final recommendations of the UNAIDS paper, which emphasises that status in order to make clear the need to retain AIDS as a global health priority and calls on countries to 'sustain and increase their financial contributions to HIV' (UNAIDS 2010b, p. 10). Given the origins and purpose of the document, it is perhaps unsurprising that even with a more balanced and nuanced approach to the relationship (discussed below), there remains a subtle but tangible asymmetry to the circular AIDS–MDGs argument that privileges the contribution of AIDS to the other MDGs over and above the inverse, mirroring the asymmetry that Katz (discussed above) identified in the CMH report.

Despite these continuities, the change in rhetoric in these documents is in some ways striking. They seek to address some of the critiques of the AIDS response and its broader developmental effects while continuing to forward the case for investment in AIDS as a key part of MDG progress. Both documents are clear that the AIDS response can no longer afford to 'operate in isolation' (and this in itself is a rather frank admission that it previously did). This is a significant shift from older narratives of AIDS exceptionalism and can be seen as a concession by the AIDS policy community to some of its critics, as well as a giving of ground vis-à-vis the wider exceptionalism of AIDS with respect to development progress. Thus the AIDS plus MDGs approach seizes an opportunity to integrate AIDS approaches into a more holistic notion of health, and subsequently to reconnect the health agenda with a broader development paradigm. In a strategic sense, this repositioning reflects the fact that there seems to be little or no choice but to harness the fortunes of the disease (not least in resource terms) to emergent issues and priorities.

Thus the AIDS plus MDGs approach does not focus solely on the beneficial spill-over effects of AIDS investment, but also places an almost equal emphasis on the 'two-way relationship' between HIV and the other MDGs, wherein AIDS can and does benefit from investment in areas such as education, gender equality, maternal health and food and nutrition, among others. The documents are replete with phrases such as 'cross-MDG synergy', 'ending AIDS isolationism', breaking down the 'artificial boundaries of a single disease', synergies which 'flow both ways' and so on. All of these phrases indicate a rhetorical shift away from the silo-based approaches to development aid, which have dominated in recent years. The AIDS plus MDGs proposal is not only 'investing in health (AIDS) for development', but is also simultaneously calling for 'investing in (other areas of) development for health'.

However, a tension arises between the rhetoric on cross-MDG synergy and a continuing (although less explicit) assumption of AIDS' exceptional status. If all of the MDGs have mutually reinforcing relationships, why start with AIDS? In theory, emphasising cross-MDG synergy could actually undermine the AIDS plus MDGs strategy. When taken to its logical conclusion (i.e. suggesting the possibility of synergy between all MDGs, not just MDG6 and the other MDGs), cross-MDG synergy provides a basis for further integrating the MDGs into a more holistic programme, rather than justifying AIDS as a starting point or the basis of a cross-cutting approach. If the aim of AIDS plus MDGs is to secure AIDS' position vis-à-vis other development issues, the logic presented seems to suggest that a similar exceptionality argument could in principle be used in support of alternative prioritisations by the advocates of, say, education or maternal health. Indeed, even more fundamentally, the emphasis on cross-MDG synergy could be read as a critique of the entire MDG project, suggesting that the approach of isolating specific issues, setting goals and targets around them, and the silo-based responses that have resulted, are to blame for MDG underachievement. The MDGs were fundamentally about the selection of a small number of development priorities. The problems inherent in that approach, which have long been discussed, are now becoming impossible to ignore. If the AIDS plus MDGs approach is accepted as evidence of a recognition of the legitimacy of this critique, then a radical restructuring of international development efforts in the post-2015 era would be the logical recommended conclusion.

However, both documents *do* proceed from an assumption that in some ways AIDS constitutes a natural starting point for understanding the relationships between all MDGs. In part this is no doubt a legacy of AIDS exceptionalism and a natural result of the mandates of the institutions behind the AIDS plus MDGs approach. But it is also the product of a view that the massive global focus on AIDS over the past decade has generated some important lessons that can be applied to other MDGs. The documents go to considerable lengths to explain the ways in which some of the key successes of the global AIDS response should pollinate approaches to the other MDGs, especially with regard to the centrality of human rights, the mobilisation of civil society and ways of galvanising political will and resources. In the words of the UNAIDS document:

> Investing strategically to address multiple MDGs, and releasing the power, capacity and innovation of the AIDS movement, may provide one of the best opportunities to 'do the MDGs' differently. (UNAIDS 2010b, p. 1)

There is also another notable shift evident in the emphasis on the demedicalisation of the AIDS response and the need to engage more broadly with the underlying social and economic determinants of health. Claiming to learn the lessons from the history of the response to AIDS, the UNDP/UNAIDS document notes the following:

> The most successful programmes have combined biomedical technologies and behavioural interventions with multi-sectoral strategies that address human rights and the underlying socio-economic conditions that render a population more vulnerable to infection. It is these multi-sectoral strategies that are at the heart of UNDP's mandate on AIDS, the new UNAIDS Outcome Framework and the MDGs themselves. (UNDP/UNAIDS 2011, p. 6)

Of course, this goes to the heart of at least 10 years of criticism of the manner in which vertical disease-specific programmes, including AIDS, have pursued heavily biomedically oriented approaches to the cost of attention to the social determinants of health. One aspect of this, the debate over the appropriate balance between treatment and prevention, has remained unabated for many years. There have been recent signs of a move back towards a greater emphasis on prevention, not least in recognition of the fact that it is increasingly evident that we cannot 'treat our way out' of the AIDS crisis. There are signs in the AIDS plus MDGs approach of this subtle shift back towards prevention, which are broadly understood:

> Exacerbating the sense of crisis has been the limited efficacy of conventional biomedical and public health approaches, the bulwarks against disease throughout the 20th century. While an expanding array of biomedical tools (e.g., condoms and antiretroviral drugs), behavioural approaches, and increasingly, structural approaches (what has been termed 'combination prevention') have yielded important progress, they have ultimately been unable to halt the epidemic's course over the past 30 years.... It is clear that health sector interventions and biomedical technologies (either existing or in development) alone are inadequate to meet the challenge of the AIDS pandemic. (UNDP/UNAIDS 2011, p. 3)

This also ties in with the critique of the short-term nature of contemporary select disease-specific approaches, and with discussions around a redefined understanding of 'sustainability', one which is based not on the goal of self-sufficiency of domestic health systems, but rather on domestic efforts being supplemented by a predictable and reliable level of international support (Ooms *et al.* 2010). In this redefinition, domestic self-sufficiency, long the sacred cow of development and health policy thinking, is treated as illusory, with international aid and health assistance being the only realistic and viable vehicle for medium-term sustainability. As Ooms *et al.* have noted (2010), the global AIDS response was to a great extent responsible for bringing about this new thinking (or reframing of what sustainability can mean), and Michel Kazatchkine, former Executive Director of the Global Fund, has been a high-profile supporter of viewing sustained international support as central to sustainability. The significant scale-up in AIDS treatment has led to millions more people receiving the drugs they need, and, as noted above, this has only been possible because of massive international investment, especially from the G8. There exists a clear (and widely recognised) ethical imperative to continue to provide these treatments to those who have begun them for the remainder of their lives. Sustaining this level of provision – even without adding to the numbers receiving treatment – will require a continued and reliable commitment from international donors. The AIDS plus MDGs approach is clearly influenced by these developments, and it explicitly seeks to make a case for a shift 'from emergency mode to a long-term response' (UNDP/UNAIDS 2011, p. 8).

The AIDS plus MDGs approach, therefore, is not merely reactive to the current political and economic context, but it is also forward-thinking, seeking to frame AIDS' relationship to development as a whole in such a way as to secure AIDS' place in the future of international development and to ensure that the global AIDS response is sustainable in the long term.

Conclusion

Here we offer some concluding thoughts that examine what the AIDS plus MDGs approach can tell us about the changing landscape of global health governance, the position of AIDS within it and the use of framing in global health. It is clear from the preceding discussion that the AIDS plus MDGs approach represents a modification of old narratives, despite building upon a well-established framing of AIDS as a development issue. Rather than being presented as *the* route for wider development and policy alleviation – with AIDS' status in global health policy and the MDGs arguably being 'exceptional' – the rhetoric of the AIDS plus MDGs approach indicates a move in the direction of 'de-exceptionalisation'. In doing so, the proponents of the AIDS plus MDGs approach appear to be strategically repositioning AIDS as part of a wider development project, stressing AIDS' dependency on broader development progress rather than merely its contribution to it.

The framers are clearly responding to a changing political and economic context, and indeed this fact is explicitly stated within the documents themselves. Awareness of the impact of the financial crisis and the waning political traction of AIDS as a priority issue vis-à-vis 'rising' health issue areas looms large over both documents. Nonetheless, also evident is a response to some of the criticisms of the AIDS response, particularly the complaints over the select disease-focused nature of the MDGs, its short-term nature, the biomedical bias of current responses and the need to escape from silo-based discrete development interventions. So what can this changing AIDS development narrative tell us about framing in global health more generally?

First, this case highlights the fact that framing is a strategic activity, used in order to forward particular claims, and often in order to secure (or in this case maintain) resources. It is also clear that the AIDS community is not only conscious of the present vulnerability of AIDS to competing priorities, but is capable of responding and adapting to that context. The MDG period has been characterised by reflection on not only the efficacy of the targets themselves, but also the ways to achieve them. Lessons have been learned from both successes and failures, not least in regard to the relationship between the three health-related MDGs and the health systems on which they depend. Attitudes within the AIDS community, in particular over the desirability of closer collaboration with other sectors, have gradually been changing and in the AIDS plus MDGs approach, are set out clearly as a forward-thinking policy proposal.

Second, frames are malleable as they often draw on contested concepts – in this case 'development' – with the meaning of the particular concept being taken as 'common sense' and obvious to a wide audience. In framing AIDS as a development issue, but doing so narrowly in relation to the MDG process, the proponents of the AIDS plus MDGs approach avoid being drawn into a convoluted debate over the meaning of 'development'. In both sections of this paper we have seen how 'development' has been represented in particular ways, leading to certain dominant policy frameworks, most notably the MDGs, setting the terrain on which interventions and action on 'development' are carried out. In the relationship between AIDS and development, the documents analysed here suggest a shift from 'AIDS to development' to 'AIDS *and* development'. Despite the rhetoric about the need to engage with broader structural determinants, the focus in practice is on the relationship with the other seven MDGs. The question remains, of course, as to whether this call for partnership and 'de-silo-isation' is merely a rhetorical strategy for securing continued resources for AIDS among other development priorities, or whether is it a genuine case of 'lessons learned'. It is too soon to tell whether the AIDS plus MDGs approach will have a genuinely transformative policy impact, despite the significant change in rhetoric. While the 'new' approach could be characterised as a rearguard action of a community feeling under siege, there are also signs that it is looking further into the future, not least in terms of the looming end of the MDG period in 2015 and ongoing discussions over future development targets.

Acknowledgements

This paper draws on insights about AIDS as a development issue gathered during interviews conducted by the authors in 2010–2011 with key individuals and organisations in London, New York, Washington, DC, and Geneva. This research has been made possible through funding from the European Research Council under the European Community's Seventh Framework Programme – Ideas Grant 230489 GHG. All views expressed in this article remain those of the authors.

References

Annan, K., 2000. *We the peoples: the role of the United Nations in the 21st century.* New York: United Nations.

Commission on Macroeconomics and Health (CMH), 2001. *Macroeconomics and health: investing in health for economic development.* Report of the Commission on Macroeconomics and Health. Geneva: WHO.

Elbe, S., 2006. Should HIV/AIDS be securitized? The ethical dilemmas of linking HIV/AIDS and security. *International Studies Quarterly,* 50 (1), 119–144.

England, R., 2008. The writing is on the wall for UNAIDS. *British Medical Journal,* 336 (7652), 1072.

Gould, B., 2009. Exploring the anomalous positive relationship between AIDS and poverty in Africa. *Geography Compass,* 3 (4), 1449–1464.

Hulme, D., 2007. The making of the Millennium Development Goals. *BWPI Working Paper* 16. Manchester: Brooks World Poverty Institute.

Ingram, I., 2009. The international political economy of global responses to HIV/AIDS. *In:* A. Kay and O.D. Williams, eds. *Global health governance: crisis, institutions and political economy.* Basingstoke, UK: Palgrave Macmillan, 81–101.

Katz, A., 2004. The Sachs Report: investing in health for economic development: or increasing the crumbs from the rich man's table? Part I. *International Journal of Health Services,* 34 (4), 751–773.

Katz, A., 2005. The Sachs report: investing in health for economic development: or increasing the crumbs from the rich man's table? Part II. *International Journal of Health Services,* 35 (1), 171–188.

Kim, J., Lutz, B., Dhaliwal, M., and O'Malley, J., 2011. The 'AIDS and MDGs' approach: what is it, why does it matter, and how do we take it forward? *Third World Quarterly,* 32 (1), 141–163.

McInnes, C. and Rushton, S., 2010. HIV, AIDS and security: where are we now? *International Affairs,* 86 (1), 225–245.

Nussbaum, MC. and Sen, A., eds. 1993. *The quality of life.* New York: Oxford University Press.

Ollila, E., 2005. Global health priorities – priorities of the wealthy? *Globalization and Health,* 1 (6), 1–6.

Ooms, G., Hill, P.S., Hammonds, R., Van Leemput, L., Assefa, Y., Miti, K., and Van Damme, W., 2010. Applying the principles of AIDS 'exceptionality' to lobal health: Challenges for global health governance. *Global Health Governance,* 4 (1), 1–9.

Prins, G., 2004. AIDS and global security. *International Affairs,* 80 (5), 931–952.

Rushton, S., 2010. Framing AIDS: aecuritization, development-ization, rights-ization. *Global Health Governance,* 4 (1), 1–17.

Shiffman, J., 2008. Has donor prioritization of HIV/AIDS displaced aid for other health issues? *Health Policy and Planning,* 23 (2), 95–100.

Shiffman, J., 2009. A social explanation for the rise and fall of global health issues. *Bulletin of the World Health Organization,* 87, 608–613.

Traub, J., 2006. *The best intentions: Kofi Annan and the UN in an Era of American Power.* London: Bloomsbury.

UNAIDS, 2010a. Media advisory: AIDS plus MDGs: delivering results towards our shared commitments. Available from: http://www.un.org/en/mdg/summit2010/pdf/20100916MA_MDG_Events_Final3.pdf [Accessed 20 December 2011].

UNAIDS, 2010b. AIDS plus MDGs: Synergies that serve people. Available from: http://data.unaids.org/pub/Report/2010/jc1998_aidsplusmdgs_en.pdf [Accessed 20 December 2011].

UNDP, 1996. *Human Development Report 1996.* Oxford: Oxford University Press.

UN General Assembly, 2000. *United Nations Millennium Declaration.* A/RES/55/2 [18 September 2000].

UNDP/UNAIDS, 2011. *The 'AIDS and MDGs' approach: what is it, why does it matter, and how do we take it forward?* New York: UNDP. Available from: http://www.unaidsrstesa.org/print/464 [Accessed 21 December 2011].

Whiteside, A., 2009. *Is AIDS exceptional?* aids2031 Working Paper No. 25. Available from: http://www.aids2031.org/pdfs/aids%20exceptionalism_paper25.pdf [Accessed 21 December 2011].

World Bank, 1993, *World Development Report 1993: investing in Health*. Washington, DC: World Bank.

The global debate over HIV-related travel restrictions: Framing and policy change

Simon Rushton

Centre for Health and International Relations (CHAIR), Department of International Politics, Aberystwyth University, Aberystwyth, UK

In 2010, the US repealed Section 212(a) of the Immigration and Nationality Act, which stated that a non-citizen determined to have a 'communicable disease of public health significance', is not admissible into the country without a waiver. This included HIV+ non-citizens. In the same year, several other countries, including China and South Korea, removed similar restrictions. This paper examines the global debate over HIV-related travel restrictions that has been ongoing since the mid-1980s and attempts to account for these recent policy changes. Entry restrictions have almost always been justified as necessary in two ways: to protect public health from the supposed threat posed by the entry of people living with HIV, and to limit the costs HIV+ migrants impose on domestic health systems. Opponents of these restrictions have consistently sought to challenge the evidence underpinning these claims and also to re-frame the issue in rights terms. However, in this paper I argue that this re-framing was not in itself sufficient to bring about policy change. Contributing to the literature on norm building and transnational advocacy both within and beyond global health, this article argues that some other crucial factors also have to be taken into account, including the changing political context (both domestic and international) and the network building strategies employed by opponents of the restrictions from 2008 onwards.

Introduction

> The world should make war against AIDS, not against people with AIDS.
> UN Secretary-General Javier Perez de Cuellar, 1 December 1998

> We talk about reducing the stigma of this disease, yet we've treated a visitor living with it as a threat. If we want to be the global leader in combating HIV/AIDS, we need to act like it.
> President Barack Obama, 30 October 2009

For over 20 years US immigration regulations stated that people living with HIV (PLWHIV) were inadmissible for entry into the country without being granted a waiver. Having formally removed that restriction in 2010 – a year designated by

UNAIDS as the 'year of equal freedom of movement for all' – the US has finally aligned itself with those countries that no longer (or in many cases never did) impose entry restrictions on PLWHIV. Other countries – including Canada, South Korea and China – have also amended their immigration regulations to address this issue in the last few years. It may be too early for those who have long opposed the imposition of such restrictions to declare victory, but for some at least there is a sense that the tide has at last begun to turn.

The debate around entry restrictions has been ongoing since the 1980s. States imposing them have generally justified them through the use of two 'frames'. The first is public health security/public safety, with the argument being made that allowing PLWHIV to enter the country exposes the domestic population to a public health risk. The second common framing is an economic one: allowing PLWHIV to enter, particularly on a long-term or permanent basis, imposes significant economic costs on the domestic health system. Whilst these framings have provided the rhetorical justification for HIV-related travel restrictions in virtually all cases, there have often been suspicions that other concerns, not least homophobia and other prejudices, have been an important (although usually unspoken) factor motivating proponents of restrictions. The opposing side in the debate has sought both to counter these economic and health security arguments directly and also to link the travel restrictions issue to broader concerns about human rights and stigmatisation. In attempting to 're-frame' the issue of travel restrictions in rights terms, advocates have utilised a wide variety of techniques including the use of individual testimony to dramatise the issue and demonstrate the human costs of travel restrictions; moral shaming, linking the imposition of restrictions by governments with prejudice and discrimination; and legal argument, claiming that such restrictions are incompatible with international human rights law. A wide range of actors, especially drawn from civil society and the UN system, have consistently sought to forward such arguments over the last 25 years in an attempt to delegitimise HIV-related travel restrictions. Indeed, to a great extent the global debate has been a static one, with opponents of restrictions consistently forwarding these same arguments, but until recently to little effect. Why, then, did the breakthrough take so long? And why now?

Framing has been widely discussed as a tool which enables advocates to apply pressure on governments for policy change. As is discussed elsewhere in this issue, frames are often described as linguistic, cognitive and symbolic devices used to identify, label, describe and interpret problems and to suggest particular ways of responding to them. In policy debates, actors often strategically use frames as a tool of persuasion, deploying them to call attention to an issue, influence other actors' perceptions of their own interests and convince them of the legitimacy/appropriateness of their preferred policy response. When they are successful in doing so, the chosen frame 'resonates with public understandings and are adopted as new ways of talking about and understanding issues', and actors will be likely to modify their behaviour accordingly (Finnemore and Sikkink 1998, p. 897). The existing literature has examined a wide range of cases in which framing has been a successful advocacy strategy, often involving sophisticated and influential transnational advocacy networks (e.g. Keck and Sikkink 1998).

In recent years, a number of scholars in global health have examined the ways in which different framings of health issues have impacted on policy debates at both the global (Shiffman and Smith 2007, Rushton 2010) and national levels (Labonté and

Gagnon 2010). Building on social constructivist work, they have sought to better understand the effects of framing on policy debates and to investigate how this interacts with a range of other factors, including the institutional and ideational environment within which these debates take place. What they have found is that the ways in which health issues are framed can have a significant impact upon prioritisations and policy outcomes, and a wide variety of factors have been identified as determining the success or failure of a particular framing including who is doing the framing, the nature of the audience they are trying to persuade, the extent to which the frame resonates with other deeply-embedded ideas, the intrinsic credibility of the frame and the prevailing political context (Shiffman and Smith 2007, p. 1370).

This article seeks to contribute to this effort to understand both the potential and the limitations of framing as an advocacy strategy in global health policy debates. Using the example of the global campaign against travel restrictions, it seeks to argue that framing a global health issue in particular ways, alongside other advocacy strategies such as coalition-building and moral shaming, can be effective. However, framing alone is not always enough to persuade states to change their policies, even where those frames seem to be convincing, appear to resonate with widely recognised norms and are forwarded over a significant period of time by a wide constellation of actors. Crucially, however, this does not mean that the years spent unsuccessfully forwarding human rights arguments against travel restrictions were wasted. One of the fundamental tenets of social constructivism (from which this paper, and the existing literature on framing, emerge) is that the environment within which states and other international actors operate (including the norms which set the standards of acceptable behaviour within that environment) is not a static and natural 'given', but rather is intersubjectively established through social interactions (Onuf 1989, Wendt 1992, 1999). In turn, the identities and interests of states are constructed through their self-understandings of their own position and role within that external environment. As Wendt, in his discussion of the relationship between 'agents' and 'structure', puts it:

> Each is in one sense an effect of the other; they are "co-determined". Social structures are the result of the intended and unintended consequences of human action, just as those actions presuppose or are mediated by an irreducible structural context (Wendt 1987, p. 360).

Thus agents, and the ideas they promote, have the potential to change the international environment, not least through the creation of new norms that alter shared understandings of the behaviour expected of states. Even when these ideas do not immediately precipitate policy change, they can play a part in gradually changing the political context and in creating a more receptive audience. In this case, the enormous efforts AIDS activists made to establish human rights as fundamental to the global response to AIDS – and to argue that travel restrictions negatively impacted upon those rights – were an important foundation on which advocates were subsequently able to build.

The paper begins by examining the campaign against HIV-related travel restrictions, arguing that it has been remarkably consistent in its arguments over time and that re-framing travel restrictions as a violation of human rights has been central to this effort. The paper then moves on to put forward some possible explanations for some of the recent high-profile examples of policy change, in the process seeking to shed light on a number of factors that, alongside framing, seem to have played a crucial role in bringing about policy change. The paper concludes with a discussion of the light that this case can shed on the use of framing in global health advocacy (and indeed advocacy more widely), in particular on the relationship between framers, their audience and the political context within which they operate.

The global debate over HIV-related travel restrictions

The imposition of HIV-related travel restrictions has usually been justified by governments (and, much less frequently, by scholars (e.g. Nelson 1987)) on two principle grounds (Cimini 1991–1992, Nieburg *et al.* 2007, pp. 5–6, Ecumenical Advocacy Alliance 2008, p. 1). The first is protecting the public against the supposed threat posed by HIV+ visitors and/or immigrants – a fear which clearly motivated many proponents of restricting entry, typified by a comment made by Pat Buchanan who asked, 'Why would you knowingly bring into this country hundreds and hundreds of people who are carriers of this infection and who could pass it on and kill American citizens' (cited in Quereshi 1995, p. 100)? Indeed, it was the addition of HIV to the list of 'dangerous contagious diseases' that brought the US entry restrictions into being in the first place. The second common justification is an economic argument that the long-term costs of providing the necessary treatment and care for PLWHIV is a burden upon the state's resources, and as such grounds on which to deny entry. This rationale was also evident at the time the US restrictions were imposed, with some being concerned that, 'people from around the world might try to get residence in the US in order to get treatment' (Laurence Farer, cited in Allin 1988, p. 1055). This rationale proved persistent; a letter, signed by 67 Republican members of the House of Representatives, opposing a proposal in 1991 to lift the US's immigration restrictions on PLWHIV, again made the case clearly

> The overall economic cost of allowing HIV infected immigrants into the US will be significant. Orange County Department of Health in California reports that .5% of all those tested pursuant to the immigration amnesty programme have tested positive for HIV, 38 individuals in all. At US$75,000 per person, that amounts to nearly US$3 million in health care costs in Orange County alone (Aids.org. n.d.).

According to UNAIDS and the IOM, this fear of an influx of treatment-seeking migrants became even more prominent from the mid-1990s on when antiretroviral treatments started to become available in developed countries but were still largely inaccessible to those in the developing world (UNAIDS/IOM 2004, p. 1).

In this section, I examine the arguments that have been put forward by those opposing travel restrictions. I trace the remarkable consistency in the arguments and frames they have deployed over time, with the essential contours of the debate having remained more or less unaltered since the mid-1980s.

The World Health Organization (WHO) made a strong case against the imposition of HIV-related travel restrictions from a very early stage in the development of the epidemic. As early as 1985, the year in which a reliable HIV test first became available, a meeting of directors of WHO collaborating centres discussed the travel restrictions issue after member states had sought the WHO's advice. The meeting concluded that testing and certification of international travellers were not warranted. As the meeting was reported in the *Weekly Epidemiological Record*, that advice appeared to be on the basis of two findings: testing and certification were not warranted on public health grounds and they were not required under the International Health Regulations (WHO 1986). From that point onwards, the lack of evidence to support the idea that travel restrictions serve a useful public health purpose has been one of the main arguments used against them both by international organisations and civil society actors. A range of flaws in the claim that travel restrictions protect public health have been identified. These include the limitations of testing technology, which means that recently infected immigrants may not be identified as HIV+ (Cimini 1991–1992, pp. 380–385, UNAIDS/IOM 2004, p. 8) (as well as raising the danger of false positives); that HIV cannot be transmitted through casual contact (UNAIDS/IOM 2004, p. 2); that there is little evidence to suggest that visitors or immigrants are any more likely than the general population to engage in risk behaviours (Public Health Service 1991) and that those countries that have decided against imposing entry restrictions have not found themselves subjected to a flood of HIV+ immigrants (Nieburg *et al.* 2007).

Indeed, the argument has often gone beyond highlighting the ineffectiveness of travel restrictions to add that they may actually be counterproductive in public health terms, creating a false sense of security (Ganczak *et al.* 2007) and dissuading would-be immigrants from undergoing testing and seeking treatment (John Bradshaw, cited in Bristol 2009). Here a link has often been made between public health efficacy and respect for rights, reflected in many of the UN system's engagements with the travel restrictions issue. Jonathan Mann, who as head of the WHO's Global Programme on AIDS was a prominent and passionate advocate of the human rights dimensions of the pandemic, laid out the case at an early stage, arguing in an address in June 1988 that travel restrictions lead to stigmatisation and discrimination, which in turn threaten public health as 'those who are concerned they might be infected will take steps to avoid detection and will avoid contact with health and social services' (Mann 1988, pp. 9–10). The evidence to support this has gradually increased over time. One of the most commonly cited examples is a 2006 survey of 1100 PLWHIV who travelled to the US which, at the time, did not allow HIV+ individuals to enter without applying for a waiver (Mahto *et al.* 2006). The study found that a majority in practice travelled to the US illegally (i.e. without a waiver and without declaring their HIV sero-status), and fearing that the discovery of ARV medication in their luggage would lead to them being denied entry, a significant minority stopped their treatment for the duration of their visit. Ironically, given the fact that protecting public health was used to justify restrictions, Mahto *et al.* (2006, p. 204) note that such unplanned interruptions to treatment pose a public health risk through the potential development of drug resistance.

There has been similarly widespread scepticism about the argument that admitting PLWHIV puts a significant economic strain upon the national health system. This scepticism has only grown as the cost of antiretroviral therapies has plummeted over the last 15 years. Here, however, the counter-argument has tended to be more nuanced. Rather than arguing that PLWHIV do not impose healthcare costs, the argument has usually been that this is not always the case and, therefore, blanket bans are inappropriate and individual assessments are required (UNAIDS/IOM 2004, p. 9). This has been supplemented by arguments that in this respect, HIV is no different than other causes of ill health and, therefore, regulations targeted specifically at HIV are not appropriate (Academia Mexicana de Derechos Humanos *et al.* 2008), and that economic considerations should be outweighed by humanitarian factors, for example, in asylum cases (UNAIDS 2006). The WHO (1988) and others (UNAIDS/ IOM 2004, p. 10) have long argued that the imposition of measures such as widespread HIV testing as part of immigration processes are disproportionately costly, particularly given the fact that PLWHIV are often (especially with the advent of more effective treatment regimens) able to make a significant economic contribution to a society for many years.

As well as critically engaging with public health and economic arguments in these ways, the opponents of travel restrictions have also deliberately sought to re-frame the issue in human rights terms. Here I briefly outline four of the most common claims that have underpinned that framing. Often these arguments are supported by reference to international human rights laws and norms. Clearly, all four arguments are linked, and they are frequently deployed together. First, the principle of freedom of movement is widely cited, and indeed UNAIDS (2010c) designated 2010 the 'year of freedom of movement for people living with HIV'. The *International Guidelines on HIV/AIDS and Human Rights* (UNAIDS 2006) similarly address the 'right to liberty of movement', noting the absence of a public health rationale for restricting movement on the basis of an individual's HIV status. Second, travel restrictions have been presented as a clear case in which the policies of many states have been discriminatory. This argument has been reflected in virtually all anti-restrictions rhetoric. Often, significantly, this has been backed-up by reference to international norms and to explicit commitments and obligations to avoid discrimination. Kyung-wha Kang, the UN's Deputy High Commissioner for Human Rights, for example, made a powerful intervention in the restrictions debate on exactly these grounds in 2008 (OHCR 2008). The UN General Assembly's 2001 Declaration of Commitment on HIV/AIDS, as part of which all states committed to removing discriminatory legislation, has also been used as a touchstone in the travel restrictions debate (Academia Mexicana de Derechos Humanos *et al.* 2008). Third, the right to privacy has often been deployed (UNAIDS/IOM 2004), particularly in cases where travellers or immi-grants are required to declare their sero-status. Even more serious privacy issues are raised by requirements for mandatory testing, which, in some cases, have been 'conducted without informing people of the test or its results, without providing counselling or confidentiality and without connecting people to HIV prevention and treatment services' (HIVtravel.org. 2008). Again international law has been used here to criticise some states' immigration regulations, for example, through the invocation of the International Covenant on Civil and Political Rights, which protects the right to privacy (Ecumenical Advocacy Alliance, 2008, p. 5). Fourth, particular attention has been paid to the rights of refugees and asylum seekers. These vulnerable groups have been subject to some of the most high-profile instances in which HIV-related travel restrictions have had serious adverse consequences on individuals. The infamous case of the US's quarantining of Haitian refugees at Guantanamo in 1993 (Johnson 1994) caused a significant outcry. Yet the United Nations High Commissioner for Refugees had made it clear in its policy guidelines as early as 1988 that refugees and asylum seekers should not be targeted for special measures regarding HIV infection and that there is no justification for screening being used to exclude HIV-positive individuals. The *International Guidelines on HIV/AIDS and Human Rights* (UNAIDS 2006) make exactly the same points.

Various institutions and organisations have made these arguments consistently over many years. Indeed, the essential outlines of all four arguments were in place from the mid to late 1980s and have barely altered, despite the massive changes that have taken place in the nature and scale of the pandemic in the intervening period. Such statements have been regularly endorsed by states in bodies such as the World Health Assembly and the UN General Assembly. But despite the unambiguous nature of these international statements and guidelines, and despite almost universal expert consensus on the ineffectiveness of restrictions (Hendricks 1990, p. 196), those restrictions have been remarkably persistent.

It is true that the majority of states that have imposed restrictions put them in place during the 1980s when far less was known about HIV and the global pandemic was less advanced. Nevertheless, it is striking that the real boom in the imposition of such restrictions came *after* the WHO's clear advice to the contrary. The academic literature of the late 1980s and early 1990s pointed to an increasing prevalence of restrictions (Duckett and Orkin 1989, Closen and Wojcik 1990, Hendricks 1990), with Nelson (1987, p. 232) arguing that a new international norm concerning the imposition of restrictions on travellers was developing as more and more states imposed them. The form that those restrictions took varied widely, including, variously, self-declaration or proof of status followed by entry subject to restrictions, through to automatic exclusion and even deportation. A 1989 global survey found that 50 countries imposed some kind of restrictions and that 32 had actually refused entry and/or deported individuals on the basis of their HIV status (Duckett and Orkin 1989). The survey found that a further 11 countries were at that stage considering introducing restrictions. The authors concluded (Duckett and Orkin, 1989, p. S251) that 'while a significant number of countries have, or claim to have, rejected travel restrictions as a measure to control the spread of HIV, an increasing number of countries are imposing such restrictions'. In 2008, UNAIDS, drawing on the Global Database on HIV-Specific Travel & Residence Restrictions,[1] reported that 59 countries denied the entry, stay or residence of HIV-positive people because of their HIV status (UNAIDS 2008, p. 7).

Thus, the number of countries imposing some kind of restrictions remained more or less stable between 1989 and 2008, at just over one in four. Recently, however, there have been some high-profile examples of countries removing their restrictions, not least the US, the People's Republic of China and South Korea, all of which occurred in 2010 and are discussed in the next section of this paper. This provides a puzzle. Given the consistency of the arguments against travel restrictions over two decades, and given that those arguments have been framed in ways which, *prima facie*, ought to be convincing, why did this series of high-profile policy changes occur when it did? The remainder of this article addresses that puzzle, putting forward some possible explanations for the recent policy changes, explanations that, it is argued, help shed some light more generally on the conditions under which framing can be a successful advocacy strategy.

A new wave of policy change?

During 2010, China, the United States and South Korea, all introduced changes in the entry restrictions they placed on PLWHIV (although in some cases they were the result of processes, which started some years earlier). This led some (e.g. Oh 2010) to hope that this may signal the beginning of a broader global trend. The US policy change, on which much of this section focuses, was by far the most high-profile, a result of both that country's status as a global leader (including in the global response to AIDS) and also the ferocity of the domestic policy debate. The US restrictions were originally introduced in 1987 and from that time onwards huge lobbying efforts were undertaken by domestic opponents of the travel ban and a series of attempts were made to change the policy. In 1990, the Centers for Disease Control and Prevention recommended that HIV should be removed from the 'dangerous contagious disease' list, and indeed it was due to be removed in 1991 until a last-minute U-turn by the Bush administration. A subsequent effort under Clinton in 1993 was defeated in Congress (Cimini 1991–1992, Macko 1995, pp. 547–552). Eventually, in 2008, George W. Bush began the process of removing the ban (Agence France-Presse 2009), a process that was completed by the Obama administration in 2009 and came into effect in January 2010. South Korea's travel restrictions were eased, specifically for those on short-term visits, at the same time as the US's, in January 2010. Whilst Korea's actions were welcomed by campaigners, some, such as Human Rights Watch's Joe Amon (2010), had concerns about continuing discriminatory measures (in particular around foreign workers who are found to be HIV positive). The Chinese government originally announced its intention to remove its ban on PLWHIV entering the country at the 2008 International AIDS Conference (China Daily 2008), although the change was not finally confirmed until April 2010, shortly after the US change came into effect and in advance of the 2010 World Expo being held in Shanghai (BBC News, 2010).[2] Senior UN figures, including UN Secretary-General Ban Ki-moon and UNAIDS Executive Director Michel Sidibé, publicly praised China's actions, with Sidibé saying 'This is yet another example of China's leadership in the AIDS response' (UNAIDS 2010a).

Here, then, we have three cases of the removal (or at least partial removal) of travel restrictions in a very short period of time, and in each case by relatively powerful states, all of which are G20 members. In this section, I put forward a number of factors which can help to explain the occurrence and timing of some of these changes. Consistently framing travel restrictions as a human rights issue, and the refutation of the economic and public health grounds for them (as discussed in the previous section), undoubtedly played a part but were not by themselves sufficient to bring about national policy changes. Rather these cases seem to have resulted from a coming together of various factors, including gradual changes in ideas (in particular about the legitimacy of discriminating against high-risk groups and the severity of the 'threat' posed by PLWHIV); the creation of a determined transnational advocacy effort from 2008 onwards; the existence of opportunities to apply pressure on governments, particularly around major events; and domestic US politics, amplified to international significance via its global leadership role.

Firstly, at least in the US case, there has clearly been a significant change in prevailing attitudes towards HIV, and indeed towards some of the groups traditionally highlighted as being 'high-risk'. From the very early days of the pandemic, HIV and AIDS have been heavily politicised and responses to them have been, in part at least, driven by a variety of non-science-based considerations including fear and prejudice. Terms such as 'gay plague' were a common feature of early public debates over AIDS (Daily Telegraph 1983). The US commentator Patrick Buchanan, previously a speechwriter for Richard Nixon, famously wrote in his newspaper column that 'The sexual revolution has begun to devour its children. And among the revolutionary vanguard, the Gay Rights activists, the mortality rate is highest and climbing' (Buchanan 1983, p. 311). Even if less stridently expressed, such views were also common in US government circles. Indeed it was not until 1987 that Ronald Reagan first used the word 'AIDS' in public, and when asked what people should do about AIDS he replied 'Just say no' (Gill 2006, p. 10). In addition to out-and-out prejudice, it is important to note, there was a degree of genuine fear about the potential effects of AIDS on individuals and society, and its potential to spread across political boundaries - fears that led to AIDS becoming associated with other cross-border infectious disease threats both new (Ebola, SARS) and old (tuberculosis, plague) in political and popular discourse alike and in works by authors such as Laurie Garrett (1994) which crossed that divide.

Nevertheless, Senator Jesse Helms, the key figure in the creation of the US's regulations through the 1987 'Helms Amendment', was often cited by advocates as evidence that the US travel restrictions were in reality based on prejudice rather than any legitimate public health or economic concerns. Helms' statements on the issue were frequently vitriolic, for example, accusing President Clinton of 'kowtowing to the arrogant and repugnant AIDS lobby and to the homosexual rights movement which feeds it' (quoted in Macko 1995, p. 552). The International AIDS Society is one example of advocates' linking of the US travel ban with Helm's own views on homosexuality, repeating his infamous statement that 'We've got to have some common sense about a disease transmitted by people deliberately engaging in unnatural acts' (Kallings and McClure 2008, p. 17).

Whilst such attitudes have not entirely disappeared, they do tend to be far less commonly found – and more quickly condemned – in contemporary political discourse in the West as compared to two decades ago. Even Helms eventually reversed his position in 2002 as the religious right in the US took up the cause of AIDS in Africa. As well as a softening of attitudes in some quarters to some higher risk groups, especially gay men, there has also been a gradual change in social attitudes in many countries towards PLWHIV, changes which have been a product partly of public health education efforts and a better understanding of the modes and risks of transmission, but which are also in part attributable to the passage of time since the emergence of HIV and AIDS as new health threats. To a great extent AIDS has become 'normalised' in the West, in the sense that it can now be treated as a public health issue rather than an exceptional threat to society (Rosenbrock et al. 2000, Whiteside 2009, pp. 6–7, Smith and Whiteside 2010). Certainly, some saw this as an important factor in the US policy change with Victoria Neilson, legal director of Immigration Equality, being quoted as saying 'I think it's a sign of changing attitudes across the board...It just seemed like more of a non-issue at this point' (Agence France-Presse 2010). Whilst such attitudinal changes have been gradual, complex and non-linear (Herek et al. 2002), generally, it seems that three decades on from the emergence of HIV/AIDS the climate in the West, and most importantly for the current argument within the US, has changed dramatically amongst both politicians and their electorates.

Secondly, the development of a more-or-less coordinated transnational advocacy effort around the travel restrictions issue was crucial. Advocacy groups, in many cases with their origins in the gay community, have been vocal opponents of HIV-related travel restrictions from the outset. Whilst many of these groups, particularly those within the US and Canada, originally focussed their efforts on lobbying their own governments, a number of high-profile organisations have also engaged in a broader global campaigning effort in an attempt to delegitimise travel restrictions on PLWHIV. Human Rights Watch has been one of the most prominent, arguing against such restrictions on human rights grounds while at the same time holding governments to account for their policies (Human Rights Watch 2007a) and documenting the effects that such restrictions have on individuals (Human Rights Watch 2007b). A host of others, including the International AIDS Society (discussed later), the Ford Foundation and the Canadian HIV/AIDS Legal Network, have also made high-profile interventions on this issue. Beyond this, as discussed earlier, there was from an early stage clear and explicit policy guidance from major global health institutions, including the WHO and more recently UNAIDS.

Whilst these efforts had been ongoing for many years, from 2007 onwards a greater sense of coherence and high-level international leadership on the issue began to be apparent. Ban Ki-moon, who began his term as UN Secretary-General in January 2007, made it known that he saw combating HIV-related stigma and discrimination as a personal mission (Agence France-Presse 2009). Ban has frequently been outspoken on the travel restrictions issue, making a number of high-profile speeches criticising countries for their discriminatory legislation (UNAIDS 2009b, 2010c). His influence was perhaps most directly seen in the case of South Korea. Although there was a well-established domestic campaign underway – perhaps most notably seen in the legal campaign mounted by Professor Benjamin Wagner (Human Rights Watch 2009) – Ban also intervened in an attempt to persuade his home country to remove their travel ban, which they did for the majority of travellers in 2010. It was subsequently reported that Ban had continued to press the South Korean government on their remaining restrictions (China Daily 2010). Helen Frary, UNAIDS' Chief of Board and UN Relations, described the extent to which this was something to which Ban is personally committed:

> It was a good example with South Korea because Ban Ki-moon never knew that they had travel restrictions, and when he found out he personally lobbied the government in Seoul and got them to change it because he said "this is outrageous". But until he was Secretary General he had never knowingly met someone who was HIV positive and he was put in a room – we have an organisation called UNPlus for UN HIV positive staff – and there was a meeting between him and them, and he still talks about it. And he was extremely emotional because he'd never met somebody. And as a result he lobbied Seoul and that's one more to cross off the list (Frary, personal communication, 3 Feb 2010).

Michel Sidibé, Executive Director of UNAIDS, has been similarly forthright on the issue and was responsible for the creation of the International Task Team on HIV-Related Travel Restrictions, which was set up by UNAIDS (with support from the Global Fund and the WHO) in 2008 in order to spearhead a major global effort for the elimination of such restrictions. The Task Team brought together a range of representatives from national governments, the UN System, civil society and the private sector (UNAIDS 2008, pp. 37–39). Many of the civil society organisations that have played a high-profile role in the global debate were represented on the Task Team, including Human Rights Watch, the Canadian HIV/AIDS Legal Network, the International AIDS Society, the Ford Foundation, the International HIV/AIDS Alliance, the Terrence Higgins Trust, the Ecumenical Advocacy Alliance and others. The Task Team carried out a number of activities including an audit of current restrictions (drawing on the HIV Travel database); a review of the evidence and the drawing up of recommendations, which were then passed on to governments and other bodies including UNAIDS' PCB and the Global Fund Board. From the outset, the Task Team was designed to perform an advocacy role, 'to galvanise attention to HIV-related travel restrictions on national, regional and international agendas, calling for and supporting efforts toward their elimination' (UNAIDS 2008, p. 35).

A key part of the Task Team's approach was what amounted to a 'naming and shaming' exercise, publishing listings of those countries that imposed restrictions. China, South Korea and the US all appeared amongst the 59 countries on the Task Team's June 2009 list (UNAIDS 2009a). The US, indeed, was found to be one of only seven countries that required 'declaration of HIV status for entry or for any length of stay and either bar HIV-positive people from entering or apply discretion concerning their entry'. The other countries in this category were Brunei Darussalam, China, Oman, Sudan, United Arab Emirates and Yemen (UNAIDS 2009a, p. 6).[3] Speaking about the effect of this shaming tactic on the US, Joe Amon of Human Rights Watch, one of the foremost commentators on the travel restrictions issue over a number of years, said of this shaming effort: 'I think it was important.... The US doesn't like to be grouped with those other states in this worst category' (Amon, personal communication, 20 Oct 2010). As noted earlier, by the time the December 2010 list was published, China and the US had been removed. Whilst it would clearly be over simplistic to attribute the removal of restrictions in those cases to a single cause, the Task Team's approach represents a clear attempt to use governments' reputational concerns to apply pressure for policy change.

Thirdly, as well as such general attempts at shaming, specific events have been strategically used by advocates as opportunities to apply pressure on particular governments. In at least two cases in recent years the influence of the International AIDS Society (IAS) has been widely credited with having a significant and direct policy impact. Given that travel restrictions directly affect the ability of PLWHIV to attend the IAS's International AIDS Conferences, the IAS has sought to use those conferences as a shaming tool and a lever for policy change (IAS 2009, p. 6). The Conferences were originally intended to alternate between France and the US, but the refusal of the US government to revoke their ban led to the cancellation of the 1992 conference, scheduled to be held in Boston, and a policy decision by the IAS to hold no further conferences in the US (or, indeed, any other country imposing such restrictions) until the restrictions had been removed. Following the US move to rescind the ban, the IAS announced in June 2009 that it would consider Washington, DC as a venue for the 2012 conference if the ban were lifted (Bristol 2009). The conference venue was confirmed following the 2010 change in US legislation.[4] The Global Fund, in no small part due to the efforts of the communities delegation on the Board, has also sought to use its influence to put pressure on governments, making a statement in 2007 that it would not hold its board meetings in countries that imposed HIV restrictions on short-term visits and specifically referring to its ongoing dialogue with China (the venue for the 16th Global Fund board meeting). The statement noted that the Chinese government was working with the Global Fund to change its national law (Global Fund 2007, p. 1). It seems clear from these cases that major events such as the International AIDS Conferences and Global Fund board meetings offer such organisations the opportunity to engage in a meaningful way with governments, and even to exert leverage over them. Again it would be over simplistic to attribute recent policy changes solely to these events, but it is clear that advocates have been able to place some national governments in a position in which they feel that their reputations are at stake. Coupled with the power of the human rights framing, this puts advocates of policy change in a potentially strong position.

Fourth, and finally, the travel restrictions case reaffirms what an important role the US can play as a global policy leader. Indeed, in this case, the US has played both positive and negative roles as its own position shifted over time. Although, as already noted, public health security and economic rationalisations were by far the most common justifications of travel restrictions, in Quereshi's 1995 study of a number of countries with restrictions, a further common argument was detected that 'Many of the countries with restrictive policies barring HIV-positive aliens have rationalised their policies by reference to those of the United States' (Quereshi 1995, p. 91). Quereshi details, in particular, statements from Vietnam, the Philippines and Indonesia, all of which pointed to the US restrictions then in force as precedent and justification for their own regulations (1995, pp.94–96). This does not mean, of course, that these countries will necessarily follow the US lead in removing their restrictions, but some believe that it is at least possible that the US policy change could ripple out across the international community. As Craig McClure, Executive Director of the IAS, said on the announcement of the US's intention to remove its restrictions: 'The US always sets the tone. This is huge not only for the people who have not been able to enter the US, but finally these laws might be overturned throughout the world' (USA Today 2008).

As the US increasingly came to see itself as a global leader in the fight against AIDS – particularly under the administration of George W. Bush who put in place the President's Emergency Plan for AIDS Relief – the anachronistic nature of the US's entry restrictions became a source of potential embarrassment, which was seized upon by the opponents of restrictions both within and outside the country. Democratic Senator John Kerry, a long-term opponent of the US's policy, argued that their continuation 'squanders our moral authority' (Bristol 2009). In a similar vein, a Center for Strategic and International Studies report argued that the US regulations were 'viewed increasingly as antiquated and incompatible with the goals and practices of the President's Emergency Plan for AIDS Relief (PEPFAR) and as a liability in ensuring effective US global leadership on HIV/AIDS' (Nieburg et al. 2007, p. 2).

Conclusion: framing is necessary, but not enough

It is too early to know whether, how quickly, or how far the US's change of policy will ripple out to other countries. The early signs seemed promising given the almost simultaneous changes in China and South Korea. Namibia also removed its restrictions in 2010, while India and Ecuador 'issued clarifications to underline that they too no longer employ such restrictions' (UNAIDS 2010b). Advocates, including Ban Ki-moon, have explicitly used the US's policy change as an example for other states to follow (UNAIDS 2009b). Yet the momentum subsequently seems to have slowed, and we have not witnessed the wave of policy change that some hoped for.

According to constructivist analyses of the emergence of new international norms (e.g. Finnemore and Sikkink 1998), the reaching of a 'tipping point' is a crucial moment in the process. Such a tipping point occurs when a 'critical mass' of 'relevant state actors' (Finnemore and Sikkink 1998, p. 895) adopt the norm, and from that point onwards a 'norm cascade' is set in train, diffusing the new standard of appropriate behaviour through international society. It is still possible that in the future we could look back upon the change in US policy as just such a tipping point in the development of an international norm against HIV-related travel restrictions, but at the time of writing the evidence for this seems somewhat thin. Whether such a tipping point has now been reached or not, an important job for norm leaders remains. As Finnemore and Sikkink (1998) argue, the proponents of a norm play a crucial role in persuading states to adopt it and, once it starts to become established, in socialising more states into that norm. This is precisely what those seeking to advocate for the removal of HIV-related travel restrictions – in effect attempting to establish an international norm against such restrictions – have been attempting to do, and will need to continue to do.

Here too this case both fits with, and contributes to, existing research on the role of 'transnational advocacy networks' in norm building, and on the factors that make their activities likely to be successful. In one of the most influential contributions to this field, Keck and Sikkink (1998) outline a number of the characteristic ways in which such networks function, and all of them have been seen in the case examined here: the deployment of information and expertise to support the case for policy change; the use of framing; the use of political leverage and attempts to hold political leaders to account (Keck and Sikkink 1998, pp. 16–25). They also offer some insights into the factors that make them more or less likely to be successful, including the characteristics of the issue itself, the nature of the advocacy network and the political context. The travel restrictions case offers some interesting lessons about advocacy strategies, and in particular, the relationship between framing and other contextual factors in precipitating domestic policy change. For one, the case examined here makes clear that providing information is not always sufficient. Even the existence of a virtually universal expert consensus on the ineffectiveness of travel restrictions did not bring about policy change in the states examined here that consensus was in place from a very early stage, but for over two decades the countries examined here persisted with their restrictions regardless. Further, it suggests that framing an issue in new ways (in this case reframing the issue in human rights terms) may play a part in persuading states to alter their stance – especially those states that are concerned with the reputational costs of failing to protect human rights – but was not in itself enough. What seems to have been crucial was, firstly, the fact that those arguments were taken up by a determined transnational advocacy movement willing and able to apply direct pressure of various kinds (moral shaming, the prestige of being able to host events and so on); and, secondly, that the political context within those countries became more conducive. But this does not mean that the first two decades of the campaign against travel restrictions were wasted. If, as constructivists argue, agents and structure are mutually constitutive (Wendt 1987), is it impossible to entirely separate agents from the political context within which they operate. Framing as an advocacy strategy, even when it does not immediately bring about policy change, might nevertheless play a part in gradually changing the political environment, opening up the space for subsequent progress on promoting the human rights of PLWHIV.

Acknowledgements

I am grateful to Joe Amon and to the reviewers of *Global Public Health* for their helpful comments on earlier versions of this paper. This research has been made possible through funding from the European Research Council under the European Community's Seventh Framework Programme – Ideas Grant 230489 GHG. All views expressed remain those of the author.

Notes

1. See http://www.hivtravel.org.
2. There was a temporary lifting of the ban for the 2008 Beijing Olympics.
3. Similarly the same report named the US as one of only 26 countries, which deport people once their HIV positive status becomes known (UNAIDS 2009a, p. 8).
4. The IAS had earlier succeeded in persuading the Canadian government to change its immigration regulations by threatening to cancel the 2006 International AIDS Conference in Toronto unless changes were made (Mellors 2008).

References

Academia Mexicana de Derechos Humanos and 343 other organisations, 2008. *Civil Society letter on HIV-related travel restrictions: addressed to the UN Missions and Heads of State in Countries with Restrictions.* Available from: http://www.ua2010.org/ru/UNGASS/Press-Centre/Signatures-as-of-5-June-to-Civil-Society-letter-on-HIV-Positive-Travel-Restrictions [Accessed 1 December 2011].

Agence France-Presse, 2009. *UN urges nations to lift HIV travel ban.* Available from: http://www.google.com/hostednews/afp/article/ALeqM5jjO8WkZTKon6BE60rzWcHJEr0Fgw [Accessed 20 October 2011].

Agence France-Presse, 2010. *Rights groups laud end of US HIV/AIDS travel ban.* Available from: http://www.aegis.com/news/afp/2010/af100101.html [Accessed 1 December 2011].

Aids.org., n.d. *HIV Travel/immigration ban: background, documentation.* Available from: http://www.aids.org/topics/hiv-travelimmigration-ban/ [Accessed 15 July 2012].

Allin, N.E., 1988. The AIDS pandemic: international travel and immigration restrictions and the World Health Organization's response. *Virginia journal of international law*, 28, 1043–1064.

Amon, J., 2010. *HIV travel bans: small steps, big gaps.* Available from: http://www.hrw.org/en/news/2010/01/11/hiv-travel-bans-small-steps-big-gaps [Accessed 1 December 2011].

BBC News, 2010. *China lifts travel restrictions for HIV carriers.* Available from: http://news.bbc.co.uk/1/hi/8647592.stm [Accessed 2 May 2011].

Bristol, N., 2009. USA looks set to repeal HIV travel ban. *The lancet*, 374 (9699), 1409.

Buchanan, P., 1983. Quoted in Randy Shilts. 2007. *And the band played on: politics, people and the AIDS epidemic.* Rev edn. New York: St. Martin's Griffin.

China Daily, 2008. *China to lift HIV/AIDS travel ban – official.* Available from: http://www.chinadaily.com.cn/china/2008-08/06/content_6906688.htm [Accessed 2 December 2011].

China Daily, 2010. *UN chief asks SKorea to lift HIV test requirement.* Available from: http://www.chinadaily.com.cn/world/2010-11/16/content_11558531.htm [Accessed 10 December 2011].

Cimini, C.N., 1991–1992. The United States policy on HIV infected aliens: is exclusion an effective solution? *Connecticut journal of international law,* 7, 367–394.

Closen, M.L. and Wojcik, M.E., 1990. International health law, international travel restrictions, and the human rights of persons with AIDS and HIV. *Touro journal of transnational law,* 1 (2), 285–205.

Daily Telegraph, 1983. 'Gay Plague' may lead to blood ban on homosexuals. *Daily Telegraph,* 2 May, p. 5.

Duckett, M. and Orkin, A.J., 1989. AIDS-related migration and travel policies and restrictions: a global survey. *AIDS,* 3 (Suppl. 1), S231–S252.

Ecumenical Advocacy Alliance, 2008. *Discrimination, isolation, denial: travel restrictions against people living with HIV.* Geneva: Ecumenical Advocacy Alliance.

Finnemore, M. and Sikkink, K., 1998. International norm dynamics and political change. *International Organization,* 52 (2), 887–917.

Ganczak, M., Barss, P., Alfaresi, F. Almazrouei, S., Muraddad, A., and Al-Maskari, F., 2007. Break the silence: HIV/AIDS knowledge, attitudes, and educational needs among Arab university students in United Arab Emirates. *Journal of adolescent health,* 40 (6), 572.e1–e8.

Garrett, L., 1994. *The coming plague: newly emerging diseases in a world out of balance.* New York: Farrar, Strauss & Giroux.

Gill, P., 2006. *Body count: how they turned AIDS into a catastrophe.* London: Profile.

Global Fund, 2007. *Statement of the Chair, Vice Chair and Executive Director of the Global Fund to fight AIDS, tuberculosis and malaria on the right to travel of people living with HIV.* Available from: http://www.theglobalfund.org/documents/board/16/StatementOnRightTo Travel.pdf [Accessed 2 December 2011].

Hendricks, A., 1990. The right of freedom of movement and the (un)lawfulness of AIDS/HIV specific travel restrictions from a European perspective. *Nordic journal of international law,* 59, 186–203.

Herek, G.M., Capitanio, J.P., and Widaman, K.F., 2002. HIV-related stigma and knowledge in the United States: prevalence and trends, 1991–1999. *American journal of public health,* 92 (3), 371–377.

HIVtravel.org., 2008. Impact of HIV-related restrictions on entry, stay and residence: personal narratives. Personal narratives gathered for the Global Task Team on HIV-related travel restrictions. Available from: http://data.unaids.org/pub/Report/2009/jc1728_narratives_en.pdf [Accessed 14 May 2011].

Human Rights Watch, 2007a. *China: stop HIV, not people living with HIV.* Available from: http://www.hrw.org/en/news/2007/11/08/china-stop-hiv-not-people-living-hiv [Accessed 3 June 2011].

Human Rights Watch, 2007b. *Chronic indifference: HIV/AIDS services for immigrants detained by the United States.* New York: Human Rights Watch. Available from: http://www.hrw.org/en/reports/2007/12/05/chronic-indifference-0 [Accessed 3 June 2011].

Human Rights Watch. 2009. *Letter to the National Human Rights Commission of Korea, 19 June 2009.* Available from: http://www.hrw.org/news/2009/06/19/letter-national-human-rights-commission-korea [Accessed 16 July 2012].

IAS, 2009. *IAS policy paper: HIV-specific travel and residence restrictions.* Available from: http://www.iasociety.org/Web/WebContent/File/ias_policy%20paper.pdf [Accessed 17 January 2010].

Johnson, C., 1994. Quarantining HIV-infected Haitians: United States' violation of international law at Guantanamo Bay. *Howard law journal,* 34 (2), 305–332.

Kallings, L. and McClure, C., 2008. *20 years of the International AIDS Society: HIV professionals working together to fight AIDS.* Geneva: International AIDS Society.

Keck, M.E. and Sikkink, K., 1998. *Activists beyond borders: advocacy networks in international politics.* Ithaca, NY: Cornell University Press.

Labonté, R. and Gagnon, M., 2010. Framing health and foreign policy: lessons for global health diplomacy. *Globalization and health,* 6 (14), 1–19.

Macko, L., 1995. Acquiring a better global vision: an argument against the United States' current exclusion of HIV-infected immigrants. *Georgetown immigration law journal*, 9, 545–564.

Mahto, M., Ponnusamy, K., Schuhwerk, M., Richens, J., Lambert, N., Wilkins, E., Churchill, D.R., Miller, R.F., and Behrens, R.H., 2006. Knowledge, attitudes and health outcomes in HIV-infected travellers to the USA. *HIV medicine*, 7 (4), 201–204.

Mann, J., 1988. *The global picture of AIDS: address to the IV International Conference on AIDS*, 12 June 1988. Stockholm, Sweden. Geneva: WHO.

Mellors, S., 2008. Comments at session on 'Travel restrictions on people living with HIV: going against the grain of human rights and public health', *XVIII International AIDS Conference*, 5 August 2008. Mexico. Available from: http://www.kaisernetwork.org/health_cast/uploaded_files/080508_ias_travel_transcript.pdf [Accessed 1 December 2010].

Nelson, L.J., 1987. Travel restrictions and the AIDS epidemic. *American journal of international law*, 81 (1), 230–236.

Nieburg, P., Morrison, J.S., Hofler, K., and Gayle, H., 2007. *Moving beyond the U.S. government policy of inadmissibility of HIV-infected noncitizens a report of the CSIS Task Force on HIV/AIDS*. Washington, DC: CSIS. Available from: http://csis.org/files/media/csis/pubs/movingbeyondinadmissibility.pdf [Accessed 1 December 2010].

Oh, K., 2010. *Is two times a trend? The U.S.and South Korea lift HIV travel restrictions. Asiacatalyst.org*. Available from: http://asiacatalyst.org/blog/2010/01/is-two-times-a-trend-the-us-and-south-korea-lift-hiv-travel-restrictions.html [Accessed 16 July 2012].

OHCR, 2008. *Lifting HIV-related travel restrictions*. Availablefromt: http://www.ohchr.org/EN/NEWSEVENTS/Pages/HIVTravelRestrictions.aspx [Accessed 2 February 2011].

Onuf, N., 1989. *World of our making*. Columbia, SC: University of South Carolina Press.

Public Health Service, 1991. Medical examination of aliens. *56 Federal Register*, 2, 484.

Quereshi, S.N., 1995. Global ostracism of HIV-positive aliens: international restrictions barring HIV-positive aliens. *Maryland journal of international law and trade*, 19, 81–120.

Rosenbrock, R., Dubois-Arber, F., Moers, M., Pinell, P., Schaeffer, D., and Setbon, M., 2000. The normalization of AIDS in Western European countries. *Social science & medicine*, 50 (11), 1607–1629.

Rushton, S., 2010. Framing AIDS: securitization, development-ization, rights-ization. *Global health governance*, 4 (1), 1–17. Available from: http://www.ghgj.org [Accessed 1 December 2011].

Shiffman, J. and Smith, S., 2007. Generation of political priority for global health initiatives: a framework and case study of maternal mortality. *The lancet*, 370, 1370–1379.

Smith, J. and Whiteside, A., 2010. The history of AIDS exceptionalism. *Journal of the international AIDS society*, 13, 47.

UNAIDS, 2006. *International guidelines on HIV/AIDS and human rights*. 2006 Consolidated version. Geneva: UNAIDS. Available from: http://data.unaids.org/Publications/IRC-pub07/jc1252-internguidelines_en.pdf [Accessed 2 February 2011].

UNAIDS, 2008. *Report of the International Task Team on HIV-related travel restrictions: findings and recommendations*. Geneva: UNAIDS. Available from: http://data.unaids.org/pub/Report/2009/jc1715_report_inter_task_team_hiv_en.pdf [Accessed 10 December 2011].

UNAIDS, 2009a. *Mapping of restrictions on the entry, stay and residence of people living with HIV*. Geneva: UNAIDS. Available from: http://www.unaids.org/en/media/unaids/contentassets/dataimport/pub/report/2009/jc1727_mapping_en.pdf [Accessed 10 December 2011].

UNAIDS, 2009b. *UN Secretary-General urges countries to follow the United States and lift travel restrictions for people living with HIV*. Available from: http://data.unaids.org/pub/PressRelease/2009/20091031_ps_travelrestrictions_sg_en.pdf [Accessed 10 December 2011].

UNAIDS, 2010a. *Press Statement: China lifts travel ban for people living with HIV*. Available from: http://www.unaids.org/en/Resources/PressCentre/Pressreleaseandstatementarchive/2010/April/20100427PSChinatravelrestrictions [Accessed 2 December 2011].

UNAIDS, 2010b. *UNAIDS calls for zero discrimination on Human Rights Day*. Available from: http://www.unaids.org/en/resources/presscentre/pressreleaseandstatementarchive/2010/december/20101210pshumanrightsday/ [Accessed 12 December 2010].

UNAIDS, 2010c. *UN Secretary-General applauds the removal of entry restrictions based on HIV status by United States of America and Republic of Korea.* Available from: http://www. unaids.org/en/resources/presscentre/featurestories/2010/january/20100104travelrestrictions/ [Accessed 5 January 2010].

UNAIDS/IOM, 2004. *UNAIDS/IOM statement on HIV/AIDS-related travel restrictions.* Geneva: UNAIDS/IOM. Available from: http://www.iom.int/jahia/webdav/site/myjahiasite/ shared/shared/mainsite/activities/health/UNAIDS_IOM_statement_travel_restrictions.pdf [Accessed 1 December 2011].

USA Today, 2008. Activists, U.N. want HIV travel restrictions erased. 8 May 2008. Available from: http://www.usatoday.com/news/world/2008-08-05-HIV-restrictions_N.htm [Accessed 1 December 2011].

Wendt, A., 1987. The agent-structure problem in international relations theory. *International Organization*, 41 (3), 335–370.

Wendt, A., 1992. Anarchy is what states make of it: the social construction of power politics. *International Organization*, 46 (2), 391–425.

Wendt, A., 1999. *Social theory of international politics.* Cambridge: Cambridge University Press.

Whiteside, A., 2009. Is AIDS exceptional? *AIDS 2031 Working Paper No.25.* Available from: http://www.aids2031.org/pdfs/aids%20exceptionalism_paper25.pdf [Accessed 16 July 2012].

WHO, 1986. International travel. *Weekly epidemiological record*, 61 (4), 27.

WHO, 1988. Statement on screening of international travellers for infection with HIV. Geneva: WHO, WHO/GPA/INF/88.3.

Making a human right to tobacco control: Expert and advocacy networks, framing and the right to health

David Reubi

Centre for Global Health Policy, School of Global Studies, University of Sussex, Brighton, UK

This article addresses the proliferation of human rights in international public health over the last 20 years by examining recent attempts at framing the global smoking epidemic as a human rights problem. Rather than advocating in favour or against human rights-based approaches, the article purports to understand how and why such approaches are being articulated and disseminated. First, it argues that the representation of the global smoking epidemic as a human rights issue has been the product of a small, international network of public health experts and lawyers: the human rights and tobacco control collective or community (HTC). The article describes in particular the HTC's membership, its style of thinking and its efforts to articulate and disseminate human rights-based approaches to tobacco control. Second, the article argues that the aim of the HTC when framing tobacco control as a human rights issue was not to generate public attention for and the political will to tackle the global smoking epidemic, as the literature on framing and human rights presupposes. Instead, as the article shows, the HTC framed tobacco control as a human rights problem to tap into the powerful, judicial monitoring and enforceability mechanisms that make up international human rights.

Introduction

Over the last 20 years, there have been an increasing number of initiatives and efforts to use the language, institutions and practices of human rights in the field of global health (Reubi 2011). HIV/AIDS was one of the first global health issues in relation to which human rights approaches were articulated, generally to protect those with HIV/AIDS from stigma and discrimination. The establishment, by Jonathan Mann, of a Human Rights Office within the WHO's Global Program on AIDS is a typical illustration of such efforts (Fee and Parry 2008, Rushton 2010, Rushton 2012). Global health activists have also employed the human rights rhetoric in relation to access to medicines. Indeed, from the celebrated South African HIV/AIDS medicines access campaign led by large, international NGOs like Oxfam and Médecins Sans Frontières to efforts by Brazilian patient groups to obtain free drug treatment for rare genetic diseases, all have explicitly appealed to the values and norms of international human rights (Olesen 2006, Petryna 2009). More recently, public health advocates have sought to frame maternal and child health as a human right issue with the hope of generating public interest and political action (Yamin and Maine 2005, Shiffman and Smith 2007).

The present article addresses this proliferation of human rights discourses in international public health by examining recent attempts at framing the global smoking epidemic as a human rights problem. Rather than advocating in favour or against human rights-based approaches like much of the literature on human rights and global health has done (e.g., Gruskin *et al.* 2005, Ferraz 2009, Schrecker *et al.* 2010, Reubi 2011), this article purports to understand how and why such approaches are being articulated and disseminated. Drawing on the literature on 'thought collectives', 'epistemic communities' and 'advocacy networks' (e.g., Fleck 1979, Hass 1992, Keck and Sikkink 1998, Mirowski and Plehwe 2009), the article first argues that the identification and description of the global smoking epidemic as a human rights issue have been the product of a small, international network of public health experts and lawyers which I term, the human rights and tobacco control collective or community (HTC). The article describes in particular the HTC's membership, its style of thinking and its efforts to articulate and disseminate human rights-based approaches to tobacco control over the last 10 years.

Second, this article argues that the HTC's use of human rights as a frame did not purport to generate attention for and a will to address a global health issue like the smoking epidemic, as much of the literature on framing and human rights tends to assume (e.g., Keck and Sikkink 1998, Jacobson and Banerjee 2005, Shiffman and Smith 2007, Rushton 2010). Instead, as the article shows, the HTC framed tobacco control as a human rights problem in order to tap into the powerful, judicial monitoring and enforceability mechanisms that make up the international human rights framework. As the article further shows, the HTC's view of human rights as powerful, judicial monitoring and enforceability mechanisms has led the network to adopt a legal definition of the right to health, thus giving lawyers an important role within the network and marginalising alternative, non-legal understandings of what human rights could be.

Before presenting this two-fold argument, the article first discusses the research methods used in this study and then traces the development of human rights-based approaches to tobacco control over the last 10 years.

Methodology

The study presented in this article is based on the meticulous collection and analysis of a large corpus of texts. The collection of this corpus followed a three-pronged approach modelled on the method developed by Bruno Latour (1988) in his analysis of the development and diffusion of pasteurisation in late nineteenth-century France. First, all the relevant articles were gathered from a literature search on human rights and tobacco control. The search was conducted using a range of keywords (tobacco, smoking, rights, litigation, etc.) on five different online databases (PubMed, Hein Online, IBSS, JStore and Web of Knowledge). Special attention was paid to three of the main journals in the fields of human rights and tobacco control: *Human Rights Quarterly, Health and Human Rights* and *Tobacco Control.*

Second, all the relevant documents (reports, guidelines, directives, pamphlets, manuals, articles, websites, minutes from meetings, etc.) were collected from key organisations in both tobacco control and human rights. These included: the World

Conference on Tobacco or Health; the WHO Tobacco Free Initiative; the WHO Health and Human Rights Unit; the Pan-American Health Organisation (PAHO); the Campaign for Tobacco Free Kids; the Framework Convention Alliance; the American Cancer Society; the Human Rights and Tobacco Control Network (HRTCN); the UN High Commissioner for Human Rights; the UN Special Rapporteur on the Right to Health; the UN Committee on Economic, Social and Cultural Rights (UN-CESCR); the Francois-Xavier Bagnoud Centre for Human Rights and Health, Harvard University; and the O'Neill Institute for National and Global Health Law, Georgetown University.

Third, in-depth, semi-structured interviews were conducted with over 70 experts and advocates in the fields of tobacco control and human rights. In addition, the author also partook in a Witness Seminar on the WHO Framework Convention on Tobacco Control (FCTC) organised by both the Wellcome Trust Centre for the History of Medicine at University College London and the WHO in February 2010 (Reynolds and Tansey 2012). Interviewees were identified on the basis of both the literature search and the collection of documents from key institutions in tobacco control and human rights. They were also identified on the basis of the Witness Seminar as well as through the snowballing method (Bauer and Gaskell 2000).

The corpus of texts thus assembled was analysed using standard content analysis methods (Latour 1988, Bauer and Gaskell 2000). The articles, documents and interviews, among other things, were examined in detail to: identify the main institutions and actors involved; understand the emergence pattern of human rights approaches in the field of tobacco control; determine the different understandings of human rights at work among the main institutions and actors; and ascertain the reasons, advantages and disadvantages for using human rights-based approaches put forward by the main institutions and actors. The analysis was streamlined and organised through the use of QSR International's NVivo 10 software for qualitative research.

The recent development of human rights-based approaches to tobacco control

From the 1970s onwards, tobacco control has been primarily framed as a public health issue (Berridge 2007, Brandt 2007). A critical aspect of this way of problematising smoking is, of course, epidemiological and biomedical. Smoking has been repeatedly portrayed as a key causal factor, both statistically and biologically, of an ever growing number of diseases. Furthermore, tobacco use has also increasingly been portrayed as one of the single, highest causes of preventable morbidity and mortality worldwide, killing more than Tuberculosis, HIV/AIDS and Malaria combined (Mathers and Loncar 2006, WHO 2009a, 2012). Another significant element of identifying and describing smoking as a public health issue has been the emphasis on the enormous costs associated with smoking in terms of medical care, loss of productivity and fire damages. Last, but not least, the framing of tobacco as a problem of public health has also involved strong moral overtones, with the smoking epidemic consistently described as the product of the greed and deceitful strategies of the transnational tobacco industry (Larsen 2008, Studlar 2008). It was this way of portraying smoking that so successfully informed the 2003 FCTC, the first public health treaty drafted and adopted under the aegis of the WHO (WHO 2009b, Mamudu et al. 2011, Reynolds and Tansey 2012).

Until the early 2000s, public health advocates did not use human rights and, specifically, the right to health together with their existing monitoring and enforceability mechanisms to advance tobacco control. At least, they did not do so in any systematic or concerted way.[1] The FCTC provides a good illustration of this dearth of human rights-based approaches in global tobacco control until recently. Indeed, aside from the preamble's reference to the right to health found in the WHO Constitution and UN treaties, human rights were absent from both the FCTC negotiation process and its final text (Taylor 2005, Dresler and Marks 2006). As Richard Daynard (2011), a prominent tobacco control advocate who participated in the negotiations, remembers:

> It is certainly true that nobody was thinking about human rights when the FCTC was being negotiated. It was simply not the vocabulary...There was of course the customary reference in the preamble to some human rights treaties...but that was not something most of us even noticed.

Today, in contrast, human rights have started to make inroads in the field of global tobacco control. Indeed, while it is too early to make any definite judgements on the extent of this transformation,[2] it is clear that the language of human rights is increasingly complementing and combining with the already established public health discourses on smoking (Daynard 2012). First, a growing number of key organisations in the fight against the smoking epidemic have adopted, funded and encouraged human rights-based approaches. Both the WHO and PAHO, for example, now endorse and promote the use of human rights norms, institutions and procedures in relation to tobacco control through the organisation of workshops and the publications of factsheets (PAHO 2006, 2008, Roses 2006, Vestal 2010). Similarly, the largest source of funding for tobacco control in developing countries, The Bloomberg Initiative for the Reduction in Tobacco Use, currently finances the work of the O'Neill Institute for National and Global Health Law on human rights and smoking (Myers 2010, Cabrera 2011, O'Neill Institute 2011a). Furthermore, in its recently published 20th anniversary issue, *Tobacco Control*, the leading academic journal in the field of global tobacco control, identified the 'human rights-based approach to tobacco control' as a 'strategic direction and emerging issue' in the field and included three papers on the topic (Daynard 2012, Dresler *et al.* 2012, Marks 2012). Second, there is an increasing number of both human rights and tobacco control advocacy groups that are currently testing whether existing human rights monitoring and enforceability mechanisms can be successfully used to advance anti-smoking policies. For example, local coalitions of lawyers and tobacco control activists have recently filed lawsuits against the governments of both India and Mexico for violation of their human right to health, arguing that they have so far failed to adopt the necessary tobacco control policies to protect their health (Cabrera and Madrazo 2010, Myers 2010, O'Neill Institute 2011b). Similarly, local human rights and health activists groups in Argentina and Brazil have started submitting reports to both the UN-CESCR and the UN Committee for the Elimination of All Forms of Discrimination against Women (UN-CEDAW), in which they accuse these States to violate their right to health by not implementing strong anti-smoking policies (O'Neill Institute 2009, 2010a, 2010b, HRTCN 2011b).

The HTC and the representation of tobacco control as a human rights problem

What I term the HTC is best understood as a hybrid between an epistemic community or thought collective and an advocacy network (cf. Fleck 1979, Hass 1992, Keck and Sikkink 1998, Mirowski and Plehwe 2009). Such collectives, communities or networks are groups of professionals with a recognised expertise in a specific domain. What makes these networks distinctive is that their members, who can come from a variety of backgrounds and disciplines, develop and share a same 'style of thinking' – a distinctive apparatus of knowledge, values, language, practices and devices, which allows the network's members to identify problems that need addressing and suggest particular explanations, analyses and solutions.

The HTC understood as such a collective, community or network began to emerge from the early 2000s onwards, but it is only more recently that efforts were made to formalise its existence and structure. A critical moment in that respect was the creation of the HRTCN in Lausanne, Switzerland, in 2008 – an organisation that 'works to advance a human rights-based approach to tobacco control' (HRTCN 2011a). The HRTCN's hundred or so members comprise most of the professionals who make up the HTC.[3] These professionals are, for the most part, either global tobacco control advocates or international human rights lawyers. Many of the tobacco control advocates work for American and international organisations active in the fight against smoking, including the American Cancer Society, the Campaign for Tobacco Free Kids, the Framework Convention Alliance and the WHO Tobacco Free Initiative. Some also work for North American universities and public health schools like the O'Neill Institute for National and Global Health Law at Georgetown University, the Masonic Cancer Center at the University of Minnesota and the Public Health Advocacy Institute at Northeastern University. It is interesting to note that many of these advocates have been active for a decade or more in the field of global tobacco control (Mamudu and Glantz 2009, Mamudu *et al.* 2011).[4] For them, human rights is a discourse that has been highly successful in other areas of global health, like HIV/AIDS and access to medicines, which they are keen to tap into. Most of the human rights lawyers who are members of the HTC work for American universities and international organisations specialising in human rights and law, including: the Francois-Xavier Bagnoud Centre for Human Rights and Health at Harvard University opened by Jonathan Mann in the early 1990s; the Wellesley College's Centres for Women; and both the WHO's and the PAHO's Human Rights and Health Units. Many of these lawyers are seasoned human rights professionals.[5] For them, tobacco control is yet another area in which they can apply the legal expertise they have developed in relation to other issues from discrimination against women and people with AIDS to the protection of children and biomedical research subjects.

The HTC's thought style is characterised by a will to frame smoking as a human rights issue associated with a belief that human rights-based approaches to tobacco control will help strengthen anti-smoking efforts. An excellent illustration of this way of conceptualising the relation between human rights and tobacco control can be found on the HRTCN (2011a) website:

> [We] believe that tobacco control is a human right and can be advanced by using a human rights-based approach.

Human rights lawyers and HTC members Carolyn Dresler and Stephen Marks' (2006) article *The Emerging Human Right to Tobacco Control* and tobacco control pioneer Judith Mackay's (2009) keynote address at the HRTCN's Mumbai meeting provide another two good examples of this style of reasoning:

> Our claim is that a human rights framework implies both norms and potential remedies that may reinforce tobacco control regulation. (Dresler and Marks 2006, p. 602)

> [There is] the need for a human rights approach to tobacco control...to advance tobacco control. (Mackay 2009)

In principle, HTC members acknowledge that human rights-based approaches to tobacco control can be based on any relevant human rights norms (e.g., Crow 2004, McIntyre 2008, Dresler *et al.* 2012). In practice, however, they generally focus on the right to health as recognised in international human rights treaties like the International Convention on Economic, Social and Cultural Rights (ICESCR), the Convention on the Elimination of all Forms of Discrimination against Women (CEDAW) and the Convention on the Rights of the Child (CRC). So, for example, Oscar Cabrera, a human rights lawyer at the O'Neill Institute and a HRTCN member, explains that 'the right to health must play a central role in any strategy that deploys human rights in advancing tobacco control' (Cabrera and Madrazo 2010, p. S291). Similarly, Dresler and Marks argue that what they call the 'human right to tobacco control' is, for the most part, 'derived from...the right to health' (2006 p. 631, cf. Dresler *et al.* 2012). The centrality given by the HTC to the right to health is because the latter is the human rights norm that is most relevant to tobacco control efforts. Indeed, according to the HTC, the right to health can be invoked: (a) to forbid States to actively contribute to the tobacco epidemic by directly or indirectly supporting the production and sale of cigarettes; and (b) to oblige States to set up and implement comprehensive tobacco control policies including prevention campaigns, public smoking bans and smoking cessation programmes. As Cabrera explains:

> The right to health can provide significant support to tobacco control policies. First and foremost, the State must respect the right to health by refraining from spreading the tobacco epidemic...State ownership of tobacco companies [for example] is problematic from this perspective...The State also has an obligation to protect people's right to health from the threat of tobacco...This obligation requires the State to regulate private parties if their activities infringe on human rights. Clear examples of measures oriented at realising this obligation are: smoking bans in public places...[and] bans on advertising and promotion of tobacco products...The state must also fulfil the right to health by implementing all the relevant measures, legislation, regulation and budgetary allocation that will be conducive to effective tobacco control regulation...[This includes:] providing health services for people afflicted by diseases stemming from tobacco use, facilitating smokers' access to cessation programmes; and prevention campaigns that inform...the...population...about the dangers associated with tobacco use. (Cabrera and Madrazo 2010, pp. S291–S292)

As the literature on thought collectives, epistemic communities and advocacy networks (Fleck 1979, Hass 1992, Keck and Sikkink 1998, Mirowski and Plehwe 2009) has suggested, such groups play a critical part in the production of many of the political truths that prevail today. The same can be said about the HTC in relation to the framing of smoking as a human rights problem over the last 10 years. To start with, its members have contributed decisively to the articulation of human rights-based approaches to tobacco control. They have mostly done so through intellectual reflection, research and debates carried out in academic or similar settings. Much of this work has involved the preparation and publication of numerous scholarly articles in which HTC members outline how human rights and, in particular, the right to health could be used to improve tobacco control. Examples include: Melissa Crow's (2005) *The human rights responsibilities of multinational tobacco companies*; Oscar Cabrera and Alejandro Madrazo's (2010) *Human rights as a tool for tobacco control in Latin America*; Ragnita De Silva de Alwis and Richard Daynard's (2011) *Defining tobacco control as an important human right and development goal*; and Carolyn Dressler, Harry Lando, Nick Schneider and Hitakshi Sehgal's (2012) *Human rights-based approach to tobacco control*. It has also involved the organisation of seminars and colloquiums at which HTC members and others examined and discussed human rights-based approaches to tobacco control. One example is a 2003 seminar on human rights and health at the Harvard School of Public Health where Carolyn Dresler, Stephen Marks and others discussed the idea of a right to tobacco control (Dresler 2011). Another illustration is the 2004 seminar funded by the Robert Wood Johnson Foundation where scholars, many of which were linked to the HTC, debated the 'opportunities, problems and prospects involved in having rights arguments play a significant role in efforts to reduce the harm associated with tobacco' (Fox and Katz 2005, p. ii1). A further two examples are the HRTCN meetings organised at both the University of Lausanne's Institute of Social and Preventive Medicine and the Tata Institute for Social Sciences in Mumbai (HRTCN 2008, 2009).

HTC members have also made important efforts to disseminate the human rights-based approaches, which they helped articulate. First, they have organised numerous workshops on the use of human rights to improve tobacco control for both human rights and anti-smoking advocates. The O'Neill Institute, for example, has conducted numerous workshops on 'shadow reporting' and 'human rights-based litigation strategies for tobacco control' in cities throughout Latin America such as Mexico City, Buenos Aires and Santiago de Chile (Cabrera 2011, O'Neill Institute 2011a). Richard Daynard's Public Health Advocacy Institute did similar work across Asia and Africa (De Silva de Alwis and Daynard 2011, De Silva de Alwis *et al.* 2011, Daynard 2012). As Daynard explains:

> We have been to something like 15 countries talking with human rights people and trying to push human rights and tobacco control people together to ... get them to include tobacco control issues in their shadow reports ... In Bangladesh, ... Vietnam ... or Beijing ... we would have these conferences and we would invite local tobacco control people there. (2011)

Second, HTC members have also sought to disseminate human rights-based approaches by producing manuals in which they explain how to organise and conduct shadow reporting or litigation strategies. One example is the O'Neill Institute's (2011b) *Litigation guide on tobacco industry strategy in Latin American courts*. Another example is human rights lawyer Ragnita De Silva de Alwis's (2008a) *Basic guidelines for shadow reporting preparation* written for the HRTCN. Third, HTC members have also disseminated their human rights-based strategies by lobbying relevant national and international human rights bodies. For example, the HRTCN organised a series of meetings in Geneva with the UN Special Rapporteur on the Right to Health, the UN-CESCR, the UN-CEDAW and the CRC Committee where it outlined why tobacco control was an important issue (Vestal 2010, Dresler 2011, Dresler *et al.* 2012).

Lawyers and the promise of powerful tools

For much of the literature on framing and human rights (e.g., Keck and Sikkink 1998, Jacobson and Banerjee 2005, Shiffman and Smith 2007, Rushton 2010, Rushton 2012), the aim of representing a specific issue as a human rights issue is to attract attention and encourage action. For example, Keck and Sikkink (1998, chapter 5) suggest that the use of a human rights frame rather than a 'development' or 'discrimination' frame was critical in drawing attention to and generating the political will to address women's rights. Similarly, Rushton (2012) argues that a human rights framework was employed with the intention of attracting attention to and changing existing travel restrictions against people living with HIV/AIDS. While a human rights framework can be exploited to generate awareness and encourage action, the HTC's use of such a framework suggests that it would be wrong to assume that this is the only possible aim when presenting an issue as a human rights one.

Indeed, for most HTC members the attraction of human rights-based approaches to tobacco control was not to attract attention to and encourage action to tackle the global smoking epidemic but to tap into the powerful, judicial monitoring and enforceability mechanisms that make up international human rights. A good illustration can be found on the HRTCN's (2011a) website, where it is explained that a 'human rights-based approach to tobacco control' is about 'utilizing the legal remedies and reporting requirements of current [human rights] treaties and conventions'. Similarly, when introducing a new forum about human rights on the major online tobacco control advocacy network Globalink, tobacco control advocate Doreen McIntyre (2008) claimed that what is 'most important' about human rights is that they 'have enforceable legal protection mechanisms that could be pursued to advance tobacco control.'

For HTC members, these monitoring and enforceability mechanisms are conceptualised as 'powerful' or 'effective tools' for the advancement of tobacco control. For example, in a speech on the importance of human rights for public health, PAHO director Mirta Roses (2006) argued that:

> Human rights instruments...[are] effective tools for the promotion and protection of health...PAHO's newest initiative in health and human rights is the issue of exposure to second hand smoke and...in this area international human rights instruments have been an underutilized but powerful mechanism that can help diminish deaths and diseases in the Americas.

Similarly, in a posting on Globalink's Human Rights Forum, Ragnita De Silva de Alwis (2008b) explained that UN human rights monitoring procedures and, in particular, the Human Rights Council's Universal Periodic Review (HPR) were 'very powerful'. This understanding is shared by Oscar Cabrera who asserts that 'human rights law is one of the most powerful legal tools that can be used' to advance tobacco control (Cabrera and Madrazo 2010, S288).

These powerful human rights tools praised and promoted by HTC members are of two types. The first one comprises the monitoring and reporting procedures for the UN human rights treaties that assert the right to health such as the ICESCR, the CEDAW and the CRC (e.g., Crow 2004, Dresler and Marks 2006, De Silva de Alwis 2008a, HRTCN 2008, 2009, Cabrera and Madrazo 2010, Dresler *et al.* 2012, Marks 2012). These procedures oblige States to regularly submit official reports on how they fulfil their human rights obligations – including their obligation to protect everyone's health – to the relevant treaty bodies. With the help of alternative, shadow reports submitted by civil society groups, the treaty bodies assess these official reports and make recommendations to States on what they can and should do to better fulfil their obligations. If States ignore these recommendations, the treaty bodies can attempt to force their hand by publicly condemning and shaming them. For HTC members, these procedures offer the possibility to submit shadow reports on how States have fulfilled and how they could better fulfil their human rights obligation to protect everyone's health in relation to tobacco control. They have used this possibility by submitting shadow reports about Brazil and Argentina to the UN-CESCR and about Argentina and Egypt to the UN-CEDAW (O'Neill Institute 2009, 2010a, 2010b, HRTCN 2011b). Each time, the treaty bodies have responded favourably, identifying tobacco as a critical issue and strongly recommending that these countries set up and implement comprehensive tobacco control policies (O'Neill Institute 2011a).

The second type of powerful tools praised and promoted by the HTC are human rights litigation strategies (e.g., Crow 2004, Dresler and Marks 2006, Gostin 2007, Cabrera and Madrazo 2010, Dresler *et al.* 2012, Marks 2012). These strategies allow individuals and civil society groups to claim their right to health against a government in a court of law. Relevant jurisdictions include both international courts like the European and Inter-American Courts of Human Rights and higher-level national courts. For HTC members, these strategies are an opportunity to advance tobacco control. Litigation can either be passive/defensive or active (Cabrera and Madrazo 2010, O'Neill Institute 2011b). Passive litigation allows individuals and civil society groups to use their right to health to defend existing tobacco control policies that the tobacco industry is challenging in a court of law on the grounds that they violate its rights to economic freedom or of speech. Active litigation allows individuals and civil society groups to use their right to health to ask a judge to force a government to pass and implement comprehensive tobacco policies. Members of the HTC have increasingly been involved in both passive and active litigation strategies in countries like Argentina, Guatemala, India, Mexico and Uruguay (Crow 2004, Cabrera and Madrazo 2010, O'Neill Institute 2011b). As the Campaign for Tobacco Free Kids director Matthew Myers (2010) explains:

> We are supporting lawyers who have filed suits in Mexico...Arguing that the right to health is a fundamental right, therefore the Mexican government's failure to fully implement the FCTC violates not only its international obligations under the FCTC but the constitutional right [to health] of citizens. We are supporting some litigation in India that is also looking at the issue of the right to health...Fundamental human rights issues. India should be obligated, in our mind, to comply under both its constitution and its international obligations. We are looking at other opportunities like those around the world.

Interestingly, the way most HTC members conflate human rights-based approaches with the use of existing monitoring and enforceability mechanisms has led them to take a legal view of the right to health and thus gives lawyers a critical role within the network. Indeed, when using these mechanisms one needs to use the right to health as defined in human rights law and jurisprudence as only this understanding of the right to health will be recognised by UN treaty bodies, international human rights courts and national courts of law. There are many signs of HTC's legal under-standing of the right to health. One is the way in which the members of the network have sought to ground the right to health in both internationally recognised legal norms such as article 12 IESCR and the jurisprudence of international human rights bodies such as the UN-CESCR's (2000) *General comment 14* on the right to health. Both Crow's (2004) paper, *Using human rights to promote global tobacco control*, and Dresler and Marks's (2006) essay, *The emerging human right to tobacco control*, are excellent illustrations of such attempts. Another sign of HTC's legal understanding of the right to health is the importance given to trained lawyers within the network – a pattern that, interestingly, seems to be common to a large number of transnational regulatory fields (Dezalay and Garth 2011, 2012). One example is the prominence accorded to highly technical presentations given by lawyers like Rangita de Silva de Alwis, Yehenew Walilegne and Benjamin Meier on 'The Human Rights Framework', 'Rights Holders' and 'Duty Bearers' at the HRCTN's first conference in Lausanne (HRTCN 2008). Another example is how HTC members explicitly recognise the importance of lawyers within the network. So, Oscar Cabrera (2011) explains that:

> You need to have the lawyers in the group so they can interpret what are the rights and what are the obligations.

This importance given to lawyers and a legal definition of the right to health has, of course, marginalised other, alternative understandings of this right within HTC. For example, the use of anthropological films to denounce the exploitative working conditions of tobacco farmers in Africa proposed by Marty Otanez (2010) or the abstruse concept of 'breathing [as] a human rights issue' put forward by tobacco control activist Robert Starkey (2009) have received very little attention within the HTC. Indeed, these alternative understandings of human rights have never really been taken up in HTC publications or discussed at HTC meetings (e.g., Crow 2004, Dressler and Marks 2006, HRTCN 2008, 2009, De Silva de Alwis *et al.* 2011, Daynard 2012).

The HTC's reasons for conceiving the human rights framework as a way to access powerful monitoring and enforceability mechanisms rather than as a way to attract attention and encourage political action are three-fold. First, there is an under-standing that there is no real need to employ human rights to draw awareness and promote action to tackle the global smoking epidemic. Indeed, as already alluded to, the public health frame that has been used from the 1970s onwards has been very successful at doing that over the last 15 years, as demonstrated by the adoption of the FCTC and the increasing funding from philanthropists like Bloomberg and Gates (Brandt 2007, WHO 2009b, Mamudu *et al.* 2011, Reynolds and Tansey 2012). Second, there is a certain scepticism as to whether the use of human rights can really be efficient in terms of raising awareness and encouraging action about tobacco control. Indeed, there is a sense among many HTC members that, when compared to famine, war, genocide or rape, tobacco control will never be among the most urgent and compelling human rights issues. As Patricia Lambert (2010), a human rights lawyer and tobacco control advocate, explains:

> There is a growing movement to see tobacco control as a human right and I think that is a good thing...But when you compare [tobacco control] to...food and water...the wars of the future...climate change...The most urgent human rights debates are not around a right to tobacco control. So we should move beyond debate and into direct action through, for example, litigation.

Third, there is a perceived need for monitoring and enforceability mechanisms in relation to tobacco control. As HTC members repeatedly argue, the FCTC does not have procedures through which States party to the convention can be forced to comply with their obligations. Already existing human rights monitoring and enforceability mechanisms, they suggest, can offer a practical alternative. As Melissa Crow, one of the first human rights lawyers to discuss the use of human rights in tobacco control, explains:

> In their present form, neither the FCTC's reporting requirements nor its dispute resolution procedures are likely to influence the conduct of governments...[The use] of implementation mechanisms employed by existing human rights institutions—including reporting requirements, individual petition procedures and advisory opinions—would enhance the likelihood of promoting compliance by [governments]. Confronted with heightened scrutiny of their conduct, [they] would have greater incentives to take their FCTC commitments seriously. (2004, pp. 220, 249)

Similarly, Carolyn Dressler, Harry Lando and other fellow HRTCN members (2012, p. 208) explain that the FCTC does not have any 'enforcement mechanisms'. One way of addressing this problem, they suggest, is by 'construct[ing] legal claims to [human] rights related to tobacco' (Dressler *et al.* 2012). Indeed, this would allow 'citizens from across the globe [to] demand effective action for tobacco control' by using the enforcement mechanisms contained in international human rights conventions (Dressler *et al.* 2012).

Conclusion

As mentioned, human rights have increasingly been used to label and interpret a variety of global health issues such as HIV/AIDS to maternal health over the last two decades (Shiffman and Smith 2007, Rushton 2010, Reubi 2011). The present article addressed this proliferation of human rights discourses in international public health by examining recent efforts to frame the tobacco epidemic as a human rights problem. More specifically, it has sought to contribute to our understanding of how and why such approaches are being articulated and disseminated.

To start with, the article stressed the critical role played by networks of expertise and advocacy in the proliferation of human rights discourses in the field of global health (Fleck 1979, Hass 1992, Keck and Sikkink 1998). More specifically, it argued that recent efforts to frame tobacco control as a problem of human rights was the product of a small, international collective, which I termed the HTC. The article described how the HTC comprises principally tobacco control advocates and human rights lawyers who believe that invoking the right to health will help strengthen anti-smoking efforts. It also described the ways in which the HTC has helped articulate and disseminate human rights-based approaches to tobacco control, from the publication of scholarly articles and how-to-do manuals to the organisation of meetings and workshops.

Furthermore, the article also emphasised the role of human rights frameworks in providing access to powerful, legal and quasi-legal tools. The existing literature on framing usually assumes that human rights-based approaches are used to attract public attention and encourage collective action (e.g., Keck and Sikkink 1998, Jacobson and Banerjee 2005, Shiffman and Smith 2007). The article showed that this assumption can be restrictive by outlining how the HTC uses such approaches to tap into human rights reporting and litigation strategies to compensate for the FCTC's lack of monitoring and enforceability mechanisms. This particular understanding of the function of human rights has led the HTC to privilege a legal definition of the right to health and grant lawyers a critical role. It has also made the language, institutions and practices of human rights a complement rather than a substitute for the public health discourses through which tobacco control has usually been framed up to this day.

Acknowledgements
First and foremost, I would like to thank the tobacco control advocates and human rights experts interviewed for this research for their interest and the time spent answering my queries. Furthermore, I thank Colin McInness, Simon Rushton, Owain Williams, Kelley Lee, Adam Kamradt-Scott and two anonymous reviewers for their helpful comments on earlier drafts of this article. I also gratefully acknowledge the financial support from the European Research Council under the European Community's Seventh Framework Programme (Ideas Grant 230489 GHG). All views expressed remain mine.

Notes

1. This assertion comes with three caveats. First, there have been instances over the last 40 years when both the tobacco industry and the anti-smoking movement have used a rhetoric or language of rights, i.e., have used linguistic expressions like 'the right to smoke' and 'the right to a smoke-free environment' as arguments in policy debates about smoking (cf. Jacobson and Soliman 2002, Berridge 2007, Brandt 2007). This, however, is quite different from the HTC's efforts to use a legally recognised and defined human right to health together with the existing national and international human rights monitoring and enforceability mechanisms. Second, some international human rights institutions had already made a link between human rights and tobacco control in the late 1990s and early 2000s (Crow 2004). In particular, the UN-CESCR has, from 1999 onwards, sometimes mentioned, both in its *General comment 14* on the right to health and in its reviews of States' reports, that information campaigns on the dangers of smoking are a measure through which states can fulfil the right to health found in article 12 ICESCR. These few mentions did not, however, amount to any systematic or concerted effort to use the right to health to improve tobacco control. Third, in 1999, the WHO Tobacco Free Initiative sought to ally with UNICEF and use the 1989 UN CRC to support its call for increased efforts in tobacco control. A two-day workshop was held and a report entitled Tobacco and the Rights of the Child was published (WHO 2001), but neither had any impact and the attempt to frame tobacco control as a children's rights issue was not pursued further (Yach 2010).
2. Some tobacco control advocates are still uncertain as to whether the language of human rights will become important in their field. As Matthew Myers (2010), the current President of the Campaign for Tobacco Free Kids which currently funds the work of human rights lawyers on smoking, explains:

I think it is too early to know whether human rights will become a powerful tool or not (...) We are testing them out (...) It's too early to know (...) Up to this time with a couple of exceptions it has not been as successful as we had hoped, but that does not mean it won't be (...) It is still a nascent discussion.

3. Members of the HRTCN include: Douglas Bettcher, Chris Bostic, Pascal Bovet, Oscar Cabrera, Richard Daynard, Rangita de Silva de Alwis, Carolyn Dresler, Tom Glynn, Patricia Lambert, Harry Lando, Judith Mackay, Hadii Mamudu, Stephen Marks, Benjamin Meier, Kathy Mulvey, Helena Nygren-Krug, Marty Otanez, Gemma Vestal and Yehenew Walilegney (HRTCN 2011a).
4. HTC members who have been involved in the field of global tobacco control for a decade or more include: Douglas Bettcher, Chris Bostic, Pascal Bovet, Richard Daynard, Patricia Lambert, Tom Glynn, Judith Mackay and Kathy Mulvey.
5. HTC members with a previous experience of the field of international human rights include: Oscar Cabrera, Rangita de Silva de Alwis, Stephen Marks, Helena Nygren-Krug and Yehenew Walilegney.

References

Bauer, M.K. and Gaskell, G., eds., 2000. *Qualitative research with text, image and sound. A practical handbook*. London: Sage.
Berridge, V., 2007. *Marketing health: smoking and the discourse of public health in Britain, 1945–2000*. Oxford: Oxford University Press.
Brandt, A., 2007. *The cigarette century: the rise, fall and deadly persistence of the product that defined America*. New York: Basic Books.
Cabrera, O.A., 2011. Phone interview with the author.
Cabrera, O.A. and Madrazo, A., 2010. Human rights as a tool for tobacco control in Latin America. *Salud Pública de México*, 52 (Suplemento 2), S288–S297.
Crow, M.E., 2004. Smokescreens and state responsibility: using human rights strategies to promote global tobacco control. *The Yale journal of international law*, 29, 209–250.
Crow, M.E., 2005. The human rights responsibilities of multinational tobacco companies. *Tobacco control*, 14 (Suppl. II), ii14–ii18.
Daynard, R., 2011. Phone interview with the author.
Daynard, R., 2012. Allying tobacco control with human rights: invited commentary. *Tobacco control*, 21, 213–214.
De Silva de Alwis, R., 2008a. *Human rights reporting: basic guidelines for shadow report preparation* [online]. Available from: http://www.globalink.org [Accessed 1 August 2011].
De Silva de Alwis, R., 2008b. *HR reporting* [online]. Available from: http://www.globalink.org [Accessed 1 August 2011].
De Silva de Alwis, R. and Daynard, R., 2011. Defining tobacco control as an important human right and development goal. *Turkish policy quarterly*, 10 (1), 113–119.
De Silva de Alwis, R., Daynard, R., and Oniang'o, R., 2011. Tobacco control as a human right and development goal in Kenya. *African journal of food, agriculture, nutrition and development*, 11 (3), 1–7.
Dezalay, Y. and Garth, B., eds., 2011. *Lawyers and the rule of law in an era of globalization*. Oxon: Routledge.
Dezalay, Y. and Garth, B., eds., 2012. *Lawyers and the construction of transnational justice*. Oxon: Routledge.
Dresler, C., 2011. Phone interview with the author.
Dresler, C., Lando, H., Schneider, N., and Sehgal, H., 2012. Human rights-based approach to tobacco control. *Tobacco control*, 21, 208–211.
Dresler, C. and Marks, S., 2006. The emerging human right to tobacco control. *Human rights quarterly*, 28 (3), 599–651.
Fee, E. and Parry, M., 2008. Jonathan Mann, HIV/AIDS, and human rights. *Journal of public health policy*, 29, 54–71.
Ferraz, O.L.M., 2009. The right to health in the courts of Brazil: worsening health inequalities? *Health and human rights*, 11 (2), 33–45.

Fleck, L., 1979. *Genesis and development of a scientific fact*. Chicago: University of Chicago Press.

Fox, B.J. and Katz, J.E., 2005. Individual and human rights in tobacco control: help or hindrance? *Tobacco control*, 14 (Suppl. II), ii1–ii2.

Gostin, L.O., 2007. The 'tobacco wars' – global litigation strategies. *Journal of American medical association*, 298 (21), 2537–2539.

Gruskin, S., Grodin, M., Anna, G., and Marks, S., eds., 2005. *Perspectives on health and human rights*. New York: Routledge.

Hass, P., 1992. Epistemic communities and international policy coordination. *International organization*, 46 (1), 1–35.

HRTCN, 2008. *Summary of the first HRTCN meeting, Lausanne, Switzerland, 1–2 August 2008* [online]. Available from: http://hrtcn.net/ [Accessed 20 July 2011].

HRTCN, 2009. *Summary of the second HRTCN meeting, Mumbai, India, 13–14 March 2009* [online]. Available from: http://hrtcn.net/[Accessed 20 July 2011].

HRTCN, 2011a. *The human rights and tobacco control network* [online]. Available from: http://hrtcn.net/ [Accessed 20 July 2011].

HRTCN, 2011b. *Tobacco control and the right to health: submission to the committee on economic, social and cultural rights, pre-sessional working group, 46th session, 23–27 May 2011* [online]. Available from: http://hrtcn.net/ [Accessed 20 July 2011].

Jacobson, P.D. and Banerjee, A., 2005. Social movements and human rights rhetoric in tobacco control. *Tobacco control*, 14 (Suppl. II), ii45–ii49.

Jacobson, P.D. and Soliman, S., 2002. Co-opting the health and human rights movement. *Journal of law, medicine and ethics*, 30, 705–715.

Keck, M.E. and Sikkink, K., 1998. *Activists beyond borders: advocacy networks in international politics*. Ithaca, NY: Cornell University Press.

Lambert, P., 2010. Interview with the author, Campaign for Tobacco Free Kids, Washington, DC.

Larsen, L.T., 2008. The political impact of science: is tobacco control science- or policy-driven? *Science and public policy*, 35 (10), 757–769.

Latour, B., 1988. *The pasteurization of France*. Cambridge, CN: Harvard University Press.

Mackay, J., 2009. Keynote address, second HRTCN meeting, Tata Institute, Mumbai, 3–14 March 2009.

Mamudu, H.M. and Glantz, S.A., 2009. Civil society and the negotiation of the framework convention on tobacco control. *Global public health*, 4 (2), 150–168.

Mamudu, H.M., Gonzalez, M.E., and Glantz, S.A., 2011. The nature, scope and development of the global tobacco control epistemic community. *American journal of public health*, 101 (11), 2044–2054.

Marks, S., 2012. Invited commentary. *Tobacco control*, 21, 212.

Mathers, C.D. and Loncar, D., 2006. Projections of global mortality and burden of disease from 2002 to 2030. *Public library of science medicine*, 3 (11), e442, 2011–2030.

McIntyre, D., 2008. *Globalink forum* [online]. Available from: http://www.globalink.org [Accessed 1 August 2011].

Mirowski, P. and Plehwe, D., eds., 2009. *The road to Mont-Pèlerin: the making of the neoliberal thought collective*. Cambridge, CN: Harvard University Press.

Myers, M., 2010. Interview with the author, Campaign for Tobacco Free Kids, Washington, DC.

Olesen, T., 2006. 'In the court of public opinion': transnational problem construction in HIV/AIDS medicine access campaign, 1998–2001. *International sociology*, 21 (1), 5–30.

O'Neill Institute, 2009. *Preventing and reducing tobacco use in Brazil: pending tasks, shadow report to the periodic report by the government of Brazil, UN Committee on Economic, Social and Cultural Rights, 42nd session* [online]. Available from: http://www.law.georgetown.edu/oneillinstitute/documents/2009-05_Shadow-Report-Brazil.pdf [Accessed 20 July 2011].

O'Neill Institute, 2010a. *Women and tobacco in Egypt: preventing and reducing the effects of tobacco consumption through information, implementation and non-discrimination, shadow report to the combined sixth and seventh periodic reports by the government of Egypt, UN Committee on the Elimination of All Forms of Discrimination against Women, 45th session* [online]. Available from: http://www.law.georgetown.edu/oneillinstitute/global-health-law/global-tobacco_control.cfm [Accessed 20 July 2011].

O'Neill Institute, 2010b. *Challenges in the prevention and reduction of women's tobacco use in Argentina, shadow report to the sixth periodic report by the government of Argentina, UN Committee on the Elimination of All Forms of Discrimination against Women, 46th session* [online]. Available from: http://www.law.georgetown.edu/oneillinstitute/global-health-law/global-tobacco_control.cfm [Accessed 20 July 2011].

O'Neill Institute, 2011a. *O'Neill Institute* [online]. Available from: http://www.law.georgetown.edu/oneill institute/global-health-law/global-tobacco_control.cfm [Accessed 20 July 2011].

O'Neill Institute, 2011b. *Tobacco industry strategy in Latin American courts: a litigation guide.* Washington, DC: O'Neill Institute for National and Global Health Law.

Otanez, M., 2010. *Video on what it is like to be a pregnant woman farming tobacco in Kenya* [online]. Available from: http://www.globalink.org [Accessed 1 August 2011].

PAHO, 2006. *Exposure to second hand smoke in the Americas: a human rights perspective.* Washington, DC: PAHO.

PAHO, 2008. *Human rights and health: persons exposed to second hand tobacco smoke.* Washington, DC: PAHO.

Petryna, A., 2009. *When experiments travel: clinical trials and the global search for human subjects.* Princeton, NJ: Princeton University Press.

Reubi, D., 2011. The promise of human rights for global health: a programmed deception? *Social science and medicine*, 73, 625–628.

Reynolds, L.A. and Tansey, E.M., eds., 2012. *WHO framework convention on tobacco control: transcript of witness seminar organized by the Wellcome Trust Centre for the History of Medicine at UCL, in collaboration with the Department of Knowledge Management and Sharing, WHO, held in Geneva, on 26 February 2010.* London: Queen Mary, University of London.

Roses, M., 2006. *Human rights instruments and standards as effective tool for the promotion and protection of health.* Presentation at Georgetown University Law Centre, Washington, DC, 13 October 2006 [online]. Available from: http://www.paho.org/English/D/Georgetown_CCenter_MRoses.htm [Accessed 20 June 2011].

Rushton, S., 2010. Framing AIDS: securitization, development-ization, rights-ization. *Global health governance*, IV (1).

Rushton, S., 2012. The global debate over HIV-related travel restrictions: Framing and policy change. *Global public health* [advance online publication]. doi: http://dx.doi.org/10.1080/17441692.2012.735249

Schrecker, T., Chapman, A., Labonté, R., and de Vogli, R., 2010. Advancing equity on the global market place: how human rights can help. *Social science & medicine*, 71, 1520–1526.

Shiffman, J. and Smith, S., 2007. Generation of political priority for global health initiatives: a framework and case study of maternal mortality. *The lancet*, 370, 1370–1379.

Starkey, R., 2009. *Breathing is a human rights issue* [online]. Available from: http://www.globalink.org [Accessed 1 August 2011].

Studlar, D., 2008. US tobacco control: public health, political economy, or morality policy? *Review of policy research*, 25 (5), 393–410.

Taylor, A., 2005. Trade, human rights and the WHO framework convention on tobacco control: just what the doctor ordered? *In*: T. Cottier, J. Pauwelyn, and E. Bürgi, eds. *Human rights and international trade.* Oxford: Oxford University Press, 322–333.

UN Committee on Economic, Social and Cultural Rights, 2000. *General comment 14: the right to the highest attainable standard of health.* Geneva: UN High Commissioner for Human Rights.

Vestal, G., 2010. Interview with the author, Tobacco Free Initiative, WHO, Geneva.

WHO, 2001. *Tobacco and the rights of the child.* Geneva: WHO.

WHO, 2009a. *Global health risks: mortality and burden of disease attributable to selected major risks.* Geneva: WHO.

WHO, 2009b. *History of the WHO framework convention on tobacco control.* Geneva: WHO.

WHO, 2012. *Mortality attributable to tobacco.* Geneva: WHO.

Yach, D., 2010. Interview with the author, Sheraton Hotel, New York.

Yamin, A.E. and Maine, D., 2005. Maternal mortality as a human rights issue: measuring compliance with international treaty obligations. *In*: S. Gruskin, M. Grodin, G. Anna, and S. Marks, eds. *Perspectives on health and human rights.* New York: Routledge, 400–438.

Framing and global health governance: Key findings

Colin McInnes[a] and Kelley Lee[b,c]

[a]Centre for Health and International Relations (CHAIR), Department of International Politics, Aberystwyth University, Aberystwyth, UK; [b]Department of Global Health and Development, Faculty of Public Health and Policy, London School of Hygiene and Tropical Medicine (LSHTM), London, UK; [c]Faculty of Health Sciences, Simon Fraser University, Vancouver, BC, Canada

Despite widespread agreement that collective action to address shared health challenges across countries is desirable and necessary, the realm of global health governance has remained highly problematic. A key reason for this is the manner in which health issues are presented ('framed'). Because multiple frames are operating simultaneously, confusion and a range of competing policy recommendations and priorities result. Drawing on the previous articles published in this Special Supplement, these key findings explore how health issues are framed, what makes a framing successful, what frames are used for and what effects framing has.

Introduction

Despite widespread agreement that collective action to address shared health challenges across countries is both desirable and necessary, global health governance (GHG) has remained highly problematic. The articles of this Special Supplement apply the concept of framing to examine this contested space of GHG. In contrast with much of the existing, and rapidly growing, analyses of GHG, our focus is on the world of ideas. We are concerned with the manner in which health issues are presented ('framed'), thereby tying them into a broader set of ideas about the world in order to obtain policy purchase and profile. We are interested in how framings open up acceptable pathways of response based upon shared understandings (or 'worldviews'). These pathways, in turn, shape GHG. In so doing, we do not deny the role of material factors (such as financial resources, power and institutional mandates) in shaping GHG. Rather, we argue *both* that the world of ideas matters by shaping the way we see, accept and understand health issues; *and* that the ideational and material interact with each other (that they are mutually constitutive). The ideational therefore needs to be understood to better comprehend the material world and vice versa. This collection, in short, attempts to restore the imbalance in much of the existing literature on GHG between the material and ideational.

Importantly, we are interested in the possibility that multiple frames operate simultaneously in global health, sometimes across issue areas and sometimes in competition within the same issue area. The significance of this is that it can lead to confusion within the space known as GHG, with no single underlying logic, and to a range of sometimes competing policy recommendations and priorities. In other words, the variety of frames we suspect to be operational reflects the lack of a single coherent narrative behind calls for action, but also creates a range of competing pathways of response. One of the key purposes of this Special Supplement has therefore been to identify the extent, and manner in which, these frames operate and their policy consequences. Specifically, as described in McInnes *et al.* (2012) we identified four key questions which are explicitly addressed in these key findings: how are health issues framed, what makes a framing successful, what are frames used for and what effect does framing have?

How are health issues framed?

All six articles successfully demonstrate that health issues have been framed in particular ways. In the first paper, Kamradt-Scott shows how medical professionals used evidence-based medicine (EBM) to identify both the risk posed by pandemic influenza, and the mitigation strategies deemed appropriate. Crucially he notes that 'from the mid-1990s onwards, EBM techniques, processes and methods have been systematically deployed in a range of national and international contexts to validate and inform pandemic influenza policy' (Kamradt-Scott 2012). Reubi (2012) also alludes to the use of EBM in tobacco control, referring to public health arguments as a powerful frame in initial opposition to smoking. Kamradt-Scott and McInnes (2012), however, identify a second frame operational in pandemic influenza, namely security, which is based on a different narrative – that of pandemic influenza as an existential threat to the state and society. Security also features as a frame in Rushton's (2012) paper on HIV/AIDS and travel restrictions, where policies of denying entry were justified on the grounds that 'allowing PLWHIV [people living with HIV] to enter the country exposes the domestic population to a public health risk'. However, Rushton also identifies an attempt at counter-framing HIV/AIDS in terms of allowing PLWHIV entry on human rights grounds. In contrast, Reubi identifies human rights being used not so much as a counter-frame in tobacco control but rather to support other framings: 'the [human rights and tobacco control community] framed tobacco control as a human rights problem in order to tap into powerful, judicial monitoring and enforceability mechanisms that make up the international human rights framework'.

While Rushton focuses on the use of human rights as a counter-frame in a specific area of HIV/AIDS policy, Woodling *et al.* (2012) identify the dominant framing of HIV/AIDS as being that of economic development. The focus of their paper however is on the ability of framings to evolve. The authors argue that for more than a decade HIV/AIDS had enjoyed a privileged position in terms of profile and funding. However, priorities seem to have been shifting in recent years, and events such as the Millennium Development Goals' (MDG) Summit in September 2010 suggested that 'AIDS-exceptionalism' was under threat. Other infectious diseases (such as malaria), non-communicable diseases and other issues, such as maternal and child health, appeared increasingly to be the focus of attention by key donors such as the US government. To counter this, the framing of HIV/AIDS as a development issue evolved to:

an approach which argues that the AIDS response (the focus of MDG6) is essential to achieving the other MDG targets by 2015…in framing AIDS in this way, the AIDS plus MDGs approach draws on (or 'resonates with') a well established narrative on the existence of a 'virtuous circle' between health and development while at the same time making some important concessions to the critics of the AIDS response. (Woodling *et al.* 2012)

Finally, Williams (2012) identifies the manner in which the economic frame dominates access to medicines and is particularly used in justifying the central issue of the patents regime:

proponents of the regime have consistently used what are often very simple economic arguments to frame strong global patents on drugs as a positive force for drug development, and ultimately for the availability of new and improved medicines in developing countries.

Although campaigners for a 'pro-access regime' have deployed counter-frames (especially human rights), Williams argues that they have not mounted a sustained campaign to undermine the dominant economic frame and that, in so doing, may have legitimised that frame by mitigating some of its more deleterious effects. Williams, however, is not alone in identifying the importance of the economic frame. Rushton argues that it has been in operation in justifying travel restrictions to PLWHIV, while Reubi alludes to it in terms of the arguments in favour of tobacco control on the grounds of 'the enormous costs associated with smoking in terms of medical care, loss of productivity and fire damage'.

These articles therefore support our initial argument that five frames – EBM, economics, human rights, security and development – are being concurrently deployed within discussions on global health. Moreover, our expectation that multiple frames can operate across more than one issue area also appears supported by these case studies: the human rights frame is apparent in tobacco control, HIV/AIDS and access to medicines; security in HIV/AIDS and pandemic influenza; and economics in access to medicines, HIV/AIDS (in the case of travel restrictions) and tobacco control. Moreover, some individual health issues demonstrate the operation of multiple frames. For example HIV/AIDS sees the human rights, security, economics and development frames in use; access to medicines sees both the economic and human rights frames deployed; and tobacco control is framed in terms of human rights, economics and EBM. What the articles further demonstrate is the extent to which there is counter-framing in GHG. In particular, Rushton identifies the use of counter-frames to overturn policies on HIV/AIDS and travel restrictions, while Williams sees human rights as a partially successful counter-frame in access to medicine. The articles also show how an additional frame can be deployed to open up new tools to support policies based on different frames (as Reubi does with tobacco control); and how frames might evolve to accommodate new developments (Woodling *et al.* on HIV/AIDS and development).

A second key conclusion, in terms of the manner in which frames are deployed, concerns agency, specifically who frames an issue? On pandemic influenza, for example, Kamradt-Scott and McInnes emphasise that the security frame did not simply arise as a feature of the issue area itself, but was socially constructed through human agency. We expected that certain types of actors would be predisposed to use certain frames, perhaps as a result of their institutional mandates or bureaucratic cultures. Different actors have different ways of seeing the world and favour the use of certain levers to achieve desired policy goals. Thus, it is perhaps not surprising that medical practitioners, supported by leading scientific journals, such as *Nature* and *The Lancet*, make the strongest case for EBM (Kamradt-Scott 2012); UNDP favoured the application of the development frame for HIV/AIDS (Woodling *et al.*); while the pharmaceutical industry and international financial and economic institutions such as the WTO support a market economics frame (Williams).

What makes a framing successful?

In framing health issues, speech acts appear to be the primary method used.[1] These include reports, articles and other written documents as well as speeches and other oral statements. Many of these are necessarily public in nature since they attempt to shape policy responses or highlight an issue. In particular, the shaming strategies used by some advocacy groups (such as those identified by Rushton) need by their very nature to be public. But what makes a speech act a successful framing in global health?

The articles suggest a number of facilitating conditions[2] for a successful framing. Not all may be necessary but we would suggest that if they are all present then a framing is likely to be successful. The first of these facilitating conditions is the power of the actor making the speech act. Power need not be political power, although the findings of this research suggest that when a politically powerful actor frames an issue, it has a greater chance of success. Rather, power may be expressed in the form of social capital either through moral authority (as seen in the role of civil society organisations in the articles by Reubi and Rushton), institutional authority (the World Bank and IMF in Williams' paper, UNDP and UNAIDS in the paper by Woodling *et al.*) or professional expertise (the medical profession in the paper by Kamradt-Scott), while Kamradt-Scott and McInnes suggest that the securitisation of pandemic influenza was assisted by the mix and extent of those framing the issue. This is linked to the need for the framer to possess a degree of recognised authority in the area and an ability to use the 'grammar' of the frame. A number of the articles also suggest that effective leadership may be useful, either in the form of an organisation (from the loose network of human rights campaigners seen in Reubi's paper to that of established international organisations in Woodling *et al.*) or individuals (for example Rushton's identification of the role of UN Secretary General Ban Ki-moon).

A second facilitating condition is the ability of frames and their agents to draw on the material world. In some cases, the link to the material world is through events. For example, the 2010 MDG summit was key to the reframing of HIV/AIDS as a development issue; the TRIPS accord was vital for the development of the pro-access regime; and the 2001 anthrax attacks, followed by SARS and then a new H5N1 outbreak, facilitated the framing of pandemic influenza as a security issue. Equally, however, other material forms can be deployed. Both Kamradt-Scott's paper on EBM, and his paper with McInnes on security, point out how quantitative studies and reports can establish a material basis underpinning a successful framing. In arguing this, we are not suggesting that the material world leads to a framing, but rather that the two are mutually constitutive: framings shape the social construction of key material events or data, while the material world provides the substance for framing.

Related to this, a third facilitating condition concerns the manner in which context can provide a receptive audience for a framing. As Rushton points out in his article on the removal of travel restrictions, the arguments did not change but the context did. In some instances the context is a material event. Kamradt-Scott and McInnes, for example, argue that despite a series of events dating back to the influenza pandemic of 1918–1919 which provided a material basis for the framing of the disease as a security issue, this had only limited impact during the cold war due to the context of an overwhelming concern of potential nuclear annihilation. It was only when this context changed with a material event (the end of the cold war) that a more receptive audience could be found for this framing. Similarly it is difficult to see tobacco control being successfully framed as a human rights issue without the signing of the WHO Framework Convention on Tobacco Control which shifted the context from the rights of the smoker to the rights of individuals to clean air. But, in other articles, framing was shown to be about the ability to resonate with what Woodling et al. describe as a 'common sense narrative'; that is, the ability to present something as natural and unobjectionable. Thus the economic framing of access to medicines is depicted as commonsensical since, without patent protection, why would pharmaceutical companies undertake expensive research and development (R&D) to produce new drugs?

Fourth, a tipping point may be required before a frame becomes accepted. Such tipping points can be the result of broad ideational changes, such as the development of EBM in the mid-1990s which then opened the way for it to become a frame for specific issue areas. Or a tipping point might be reached because of material events. Rushton, for example, speculates whether the change in US policy on travel restrictions may represent such a tipping point, while Kamradt-Scott and McInnes identify a period around 2003–2005 when, following both heightened concerns about bioterrorism after 9/11 and a further outbreak of H5N1, pandemic influenza became securitised.

Finally, the continued success of a frame may depend upon its ability to adapt to changing contexts, as Woodling et al. demonstrate. In particular the contested nature of the majority of frames operating in global health would suggest the potential for malleability, allowing different aspects or interpretations of a frame to be foregrounded as contexts shift.

What are frames used for?

The first article in this Special Supplement introduced frames as instrumental. This means that they are not unintended or natural, nor are they value-neutral analyses of an external reality. Rather, they are deliberately deployed for some purpose, usually to create or maintain a pathway of response to a particular health issue area. But as this collection has demonstrated, there are a number of uses to which frames can be put in order to achieve this purpose.

Most obviously, our research has found that framing can be strategically used to introduce, undermine or change policy. This is especially so in the case of pandemic influenza. Both the EBM and security frames were used to draw attention to the issue and suggest potential policy routes. Rushton, however, shows how framing – or, more precisely, counter-framing – can be used to change policy. More generally, framing can be used to establish a regime; that is, a series of broadly coherent policies, practices and institutional arrangements underpinned by a common rationale. This is seen in Williams' paper on the role of the economic frame in influencing policies on access to medicines, and in the way in which EBM shaped, 'not only pandemic influenza policy, but also the world's influenza governance arrangements and institutions' (Kamradt-Scott 2012).

Framing can also be used to create or maintain a higher level profile in the policy world. The use of the security frame for pandemic influenza was to highlight it as an issue requiring greater attention, while Woodling *et al.* found that the reframing of HIV/AIDS as a development issue was to maintain its position of pre-eminence:

> the degree of prioritisation which AIDS has enjoyed over the last 15 years [is because] the AIDS policy community have been particularly successful at framing and re-framing the issue at various times and in various ways to capture high level political attention.

Reubi, however, demonstrates that the use of the human rights frame in tobacco control was not to retain or elevate attention, following the signing of the Framework Convention on Tobacco Control (FCTC), but instead to 'tap into the powerful, judicial monitoring and enforceability mechanisms that make up international human rights'. In other words, it was to legitimise the use of a new range of legally based tools. In a slightly different manner, the EBM frame was used to legitimise both certain types of responses to pandemic influenza as 'proven' to be effective, and the authority of the medical profession as the generators of such types of evidence.

What effects does framing have?

Frames are, therefore, used in different ways to create pathways for response, but do they create different responses? The answer to this question is crucial for our understanding of the prospects for effective GHG because, if they do, the coexistence of multiple frames may lead to different and/or competing responses to health issue areas.

The answer to this question appears to be that different frames *do* tend to lead to different policy decisions. Kamradt-Scott, for example, demonstrates how EBM led to a preference for pharmaceutical-based interventions to combat pandemic influenza globally, not least because alternative solutions (such as socioeconomically derived interventions) are not easily quantifiable in terms of inputs and outcomes. Implicit in this analysis is that a different frame – for example that of development – may have led to different policy responses focusing perhaps on so-called upstream causes of disease.

The second article in this Supplement, on pandemic influenza, demonstrates how different frames can sometimes lead to overlapping policy responses. As with EBM, the security frame identifies the importance of pharmaceutical-based interventions for pandemic influenza, but with the emphasis on deploying drugs to preserve human life at the *national* level, including ensuring access to vaccines and anti-viral drugs via government controlled stockpiling and distribution. Thus, both frames supported pharmaceutical-based policy interventions, but how drugs would be acquired and used to address an influenza outbreak was different under each frame. However, the security frame also emphasised the role of planning, preparedness and resilience, especially at the national level, and the importance of establishing emergency laws and protocols. The clearest case, however, where the security frame established a different policy to that of another frame is seen in Rushton's paper. Travel restrictions for people living with HIV (PLWHIV) were legitimated through the use of security and economic frames, while the deployment of a human rights frame was a necessary (although not a sufficient) condition to overturn this legislation in the USA and two other states. The tension between human rights and economics is also apparent in the paper on access to medicines, where the patents regime was a product of framing the issue in terms of market economics. In contrast, a human rights frame would have placed a higher value on access to medicines by key population groups, over the rights of pharmaceutical companies to derive financial rewards from investing in R&D.

Our findings highlight two further important effects of framing on policy and GHG. First, Woodling *et al.* show how an issue may need to 'buy into' a dominant frame to ensure that it retains its priority. Specifically, the authors demonstrate how, when the privileged position of HIV/AIDS in terms of funding was threatened, AIDS activists responded by emphasising the diseases' significance in terms of the dominant frame, namely development. And, finally, Reubi demonstrates how different frames may act in complementary manners towards the same policy end. For Reubi, the use of the human rights frame was to support other framings, rather than compete with them, in advocating the implementation of tobacco control measures and thereby reinforce GHG via the FCTC.

Conclusion

This Special Supplement argues for the need to better understand the role of framing in the challenge of strengthening GHG. While many existing analyses remain focused on developing better technical interventions, or 'fixing' administrative or institutional arrangements deemed flawed or inefficient, we argue that the presence of diverse, and often competing, frames act as a deeper causal factor for many of the problems confronting GHG. It is this multiplicity of frames, operating within and across global health issue areas, that has led to the crowded and contested GHG landscape that we see today.

The articles in this Special Supplement add to a small but growing body of scholarly work that seeks to demonstrate how frames are used in a variety of ways in global health to establish pathways of response. Most importantly for the future prospects for GHG, our findings demonstrate how different framings not only lead to a variety of narratives, thereby compromising the potential for GHG to possess a coherent underlying logic, but that it can also lead to competing pathways and policy responses. We therefore conclude that the presence of these different frames contributes to a confused institutional landscape and policy space where contradictions and competition are rife.

Acknowledgements

This research has been made possible through funding from the European Research Council under the European Community's Seventh Framework Programme – Ideas Grant 230489 GHG. All views expressed remain those of the authors.

Notes

1. Michael Williams (2003), for example, argues that speech acts need not be the only method by which an issue is framed. For Williams, visual representations including televised acts (such as the terrorist attacks of 9/11) may also be significant. In a related vein, David Campbell (2008) has identified how the 'visuals' of HIV have been important in constructing our understanding of the disease.
2. The term 'facilitating conditions' is from Buzan *et al.* (1998), but similar terms are common in much of the literature on the processes whereby issues are constructed or framed.

References

Buzan, B., Waever, O., and de Wilde, J., 1998. *Security: a new framework for analysis.* Boulder, Colorado: Lynne Rienner.

Campbell, D., 2008. The visual economy of HIV/AIDS as a security issue. *AIDS, Security and Conflict Initiative Research Report No. 18* [online]. Available from: http://asci.researchhub. ssrc.org/working-papers/Visual%20Economy%20of%20HIV%20AIDS.pdf [Accessed 27 May 2010].

Kamradt-Scott, A., 2012. Evidence-based medicine and the governance of pandemic influenza. *Global Public Health* [advance online publication]. doi: 10.1080/17441692.2012. 728239

Kamradt-Scott, A., and McInnes, C., 2012. The securitisation of pandemic influenza: framing, security and public policy. *Global public health.* doi: 10.1080/17441692.2012.725752

McInnes, C., Kamradt-Scott, A., Lee, K., Reubi, D., Roemer-Mahler, A., Rushton, S., Williams, O.D., and Woodling, M., 2012. Framing global health: the governance challenge. *Global Public Health* [advance online publication]. doi: 10.1080/17441692.2012.733949

Reubi, D., 2012. Making a human right to tobacco control: expert and advocacy networks, framing and the right to health. *Global Public Health* [advance online publication]. doi: 10.1080/17441692.2012.733948

Rushton, S., 2012. The global debate over HIV-related travel restrictions: framing and policy change. *Global Public Health* [advance online publication]. doi: 10.1080/17441692.2012. 735249

Williams, M.C., 2003. Words, images, enemies: securitization and international politics. *International Studies Quarterly*, 47, 511–531.

Williams, O.D., 2012. Access to medicines, market failure and market intervention: a tale of two regimes. *Global Public Health* [advance online publication]. doi: 10.1080/17441692. 2012.725753

Woodling, M., Williams, O.D., and Rushton, S., 2012. New life in old frames: HIV, development and the 'AIDS plus MDGs' approach. *Global Public Health* [advance online publication]. doi: 10.1080/17441692.2012.728238

Index